PRAISE FOR *INVISIBLE VISION*
BY ROY WESLEY

"Newton Wesley has found a sensitive and sympathetic, but not entirely uncritical, biographer in his son Roy. Well-researched and always conscious of its broader context, *Invisible Vision* is an inspiring story."

—**Thomas Hamm**, PhD, Professor of History, Curator of the Quaker Collection and Director of Special Collections at Earlham College

"An intriguing biography of the life of Dr. Newton K. Wesley. A must-read for anyone interested in optometry, eyecare, contact lenses and US History during the pre- and post-WWII era. The biography is timely in that it recounts the fact that the infant Newton Wesley survived the influenza pandemic of 1918 after being born in a lumber camp in Oregon. He and his young family were required to relocate to an internment/prison camp in May 1942 which reminds us of the harshness of racism at that time. The impact of his educational opportunity at Earlham College and his subsequent trip to Chicago where he was diagnosed with keratoconus were both impactful in his life's work. The book details Dr. Wesley's pioneering work in contact lenses, indeed the very inclusion of the term in the dictionary, as well as developing many of the instruments utilized to advance Contact Lens studies. It further details his understanding of the importance of the relationship between the curvature of the human eye, the tear layers and the success of fitting contact lenses for maximum health, comfort and improvement of vision. The book chronicles how Dr. Wesley built successful businesses, including Wesley-Jessen, after starting in the basement of his home in Chicago, to having national and international locations and factories with hundreds of employees during the manufacturing revolution."

—**Dr. Mark K. Colip**, OD, President Illinois College of Optometry

INVISIBLE
VISION

INVISIBLE VISION

*The hidden story of Dr. Newton K. Wesley,
American contact lens pioneer*

Roy Wesley

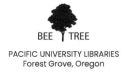

BEE TREE

PACIFIC UNIVERSITY LIBRARIES
Forest Grove, Oregon

Invisible Vision

Published by Pacific University Libraries 2021

ISBN 978-1-945398-05-6 (pbk)
ISBN 978-1-945398-07-0 (cloth)
ISBN 978-1-945398-08-7 (ebook)

Pacific University Libraries
2043 College Way
Forest Grove, Oregon 97116

lib.pacificu.edu

Published in the United States of America
Set in Georgia

Cover images licensed from iStock

Bee Tree Books
An imprint of the Pacific University Libraries

The "Bee Tree", an iconic ivy-covered tree that stood on the Pacific University campus for many years, was already old and hollow when pioneer Tabitha Brown arrived in Oregon in 1846. Mrs. Brown started a home for orphans that would grow into Pacific University. According to the Forest Grove *News-Times*, the tree was "said to have housed a swarm of bees who furnished the little old lady with honey which she sold to buy provisions for her orphan children."

TABLE OF CONTENTS

Acknowledgements, *ix*
Foreword, *xi*
Prologue, *xiii*

CHAPTER 1. Origins, *1*

CHAPTER 2. The Road to North Pacific College of Optometry, *11*

CHAPTER 3. World War II, *19*

CHAPTER 4. Personal Freedom Plans, *27*

CHAPTER 5. Earlham College, *34*

CHAPTER 6. Starting Over, *50*

CHAPTER 7. Business Building in Chicago, *62*

CHAPTER 8. Development of Wesley Jessen, *72*

CHAPTER 9. Company Components, *88*

CHAPTER 10. NERF and the First International Contact Lens Congress, *118*

CHAPTER 11. Orthokeratology and Myopia Control, *136*

CHAPTER 12. Epilogue, *139*

References, *149*
Appendix, *155*

ACKNOWLEDGEMENTS

Writing *Invisible Vision* was a tedious, arduous, solitary, and repetitive process requiring many years of patience on the part of family and friends. I am grateful for the constant love, support, and encouragement of my husband, Mark Weber. In particular, I appreciate his positive attitude as I discovered new facts and tidbits of information concerning people and stories which he heard over and over. His ability to be a good listener and motivator kept me going.

I am thankful for the emotional and moral support of our children, Royce and Craig, and their families, my late brother, Lee and his wife Vicki and their families, and from my extended family: Newton, Sandra, Morgan, Shona, Justine, Jenna, and Taylor, as well as from my former wife, Jane.

I am grateful for those at Earlham College for useful discussions and corrections: Professor Thomas Hamm, Dyron Dabney, Rod Waltz, and Neal Baker. I appreciate Illinois College of Optometry President Mark Colip for corrections and readings.

Michael Jessen for helpful conversations and materials from his collection, Janet and Joseph Cinefro, Cheryl and Robert Cinefro for conversations concerning their father Joseph Cinefro, Vice President of WJ.

Jim Moritz, a WJ regional manager who became VP of New Business Development, organized the WJ 2018 Reunion to which he invited me following Roi Parris' kind promptings and continued support (she was EDP and IT manager) and a long time employee. Karen Bruder, manager of Sales Training, for sending me her collection of WJ training manuals and materials which will be deposited at the Contact Lens Museum, Forest Grove, Oregon. To the many colleagues at Wesley-Jessen and the WJ Reunion who helped give me insights into their WJ stories.

Dean Isaac Gilman and staff at Pacific University Libraries for guiding the publication of this book and to PUCO Dean Fraser Horn and staff for invaluable support during the process, as well as to former Dean Jennifer Coyle.

FOREWORD

As young students in the 1970s we were introduced to the name Newton Wesley as part of our contact lens education; often as it referred to the Wesley-Jessen Company of Chicago, Illinois where many of the contact lenses we were learning to use were fabricated. Little did we know then that this "larger-than-life" man would be instrumental in creating the global contact lens market we have today. As contact lens historians, we are aware of the many stories regarding the people involved in the development of our industry, and those of Dr. Wesley are no exception, however there is so much more in this compelling book.

From a son's perspective, Roy Wesley takes us through the fascinating story of his father, whose creativity and entrepreneurial spirt were shaped by the political, social, and economic events of his time. Roy's fascinating narrative intertwines his family's experiences throughout the major events of the twentieth century including the Great Depression, World War II, and the post-war years.

The story weaves from the Pacific Northwest to the Midwest and finally, around the globe. It chronicles a man who attends, purchases, and then sells an optometry college, all before the age of thirty. It continues with Newton becoming an academic, inventor, clinician, promoter, and businessman. It even includes a US presidential candidate listing the purchase and sale of a company with the Wesley name on it at the top of his investment accomplishments. And—there's so much more.

Writing a biography cannot be easy under any circumstances. This must be especially so if it's about a family member, in particular a parent. In *Invisible Vision*, the Wesley family story comes to life through the eyes and words of Roy Wesley. At times, Roy describes his father from an author's perspective, simply stating the facts. Elsewhere, he's the little boy son, describing in wonderment being in the cockpit of Dad's twin Beech airplane, so proud that he's being made to feel as if he's the one piloting.

We found the entire book to be extremely interesting and

insightful. It documents one man's journey, while taking us through the development of a device that is worn by millions of people throughout the world. We compliment Roy Wesley for bringing to life his father's story to current and future generations of those interested in better understanding the human characteristics of drive, perseverance, and a reverence for life.

For 65 years (1946-2011), the field of contact lenses was dramatically influenced by Newton Wesley. Even today, his impact continues to be present in almost every discipline within our industry from lens design and materials to manufacturing and of course... marketing. His story and life achievements illustrate how a single-minded individual can change the entire trajectory of a global industry by creating a market where essentially none existed and making the term "contact lenses" a household word. His legacy and footprint on our industry will be forever remembered in the archives of contact lens history.

Patrick J. Caroline and Craig W. Norman
Curators of the Contact Lens Museum in Forest Grove, Oregon

PROLOGUE

Sight is the most important of our five senses. We gather most of our information about the world around us through our eyes. It is the sense we take most often for granted. Contact lenses create a form of invisible vision. These small items are unseen by others and unnoticed by the wearer when doing their job correctly. When vision is lost or imperfect, this critical faculty can not be ignored. *Invisible Vision* traces the history of Dr. Newton K. Wesley's contributions to the creation and development of contact lenses in the United States and internationally.

The survival of the human species depends on vision. We need to see to gather and prepare food, to be wary of predators, to take care of our daily functions. The natural course of evolution selected for good eyesight. In the past, Darwinism eliminated those who did not see well, while survivors continued to pass on their good genes. Humans are no longer outdoor creatures foraging, hunting, or roaming through forests and plains. We have moved our lifestyle indoors, which creates new demands on our near vision skills: reading books, papers, computers, mobile phones. Artificial lighting, the lack of sunshine, fresh air, and active mobility have begun to compromise our distance vision. Over 40% of Americans are near-sighted (myopic) and is trending toward 50% within the 21st century. In Asia, 80%-90% of the population is already near-sighted.

Glasses have been the traditional method of vision correction since the 13th century. An alternative, contact lenses, appeared at the end of the 19th century. Today almost all of us know about contact lenses as a method of improving vision or altering eye color. More dramatically, cosmetic contacts might complete a Halloween costume. When we think of contact lenses for vision improvement, we hardly notice those among us who are wearing them because, unlike glasses, they are invisible. It is not a product that sells itself. Someone wearing glasses may hear, "Where did you get those great frames? I would love a pair like that." That is not the experience of an average contact lens wearer. Contact lenses solve many vision problems:

- Myopia (near-sightedness)
- Hyperopia (far-sightedness)
- Astigmatism (distortion caused by an irregular curvature of the cornea or the interior lens)
- Presbyopia (the need for correction when reading)

Contact lenses float on the tear layer of the eye. The closer the lens is to the eye, the more accurate the image of the world. Technically, this defines the vertex distance, the distance between the back surface of a corrective lens to the eye. When the vertex distance is zero, as in a contact lens, there is no distortion. Glasses sit 12 to 14 mm from the eye. Medium to high prescriptions can distort vision unless corrected for the change.

Contact lenses give clear, unobstructed peripheral vision compared with spectacles because there is no frame to obstruct side vision. Contacts provide the best correction for eye diseases such as keratoconus and aniseikonia (unequal images between the eyes).

Marketing a new product often depends on a visual presentation that creates demand. We need something tangible that says "Buy me" or creates an urge to own something that gives status and acceptance with friends and neighbors. This fundamental problem confronted a young Newton Wesley when he and George Jessen began their fledgling contact lens business, Wesley-Jessen, in the mid-1940s. There was no ready market for the product at that time. Even worse, there was not even a public awareness that such a product could help people see without glasses. Why and how did Dr. Wesley manage to create and develop contact lenses from an unknown product to a nationally and globally desired consumer product? Federal and state regulations required contact lenses to be sold to licensed doctors and not directly to consumers. This requirement made the manufacturers virtually invisible to the public.

During the 1930s to 1940s, contact lenses were not a household word. At the time, the eye devices were known as corneal lenses or scleral lenses. Eye care professionals treated eyes disfigured by accidents or congenital problems with scleral lenses. Eyes afflicted by corneal diseases such as keratoconus received consideration for corneal lens treatment. For the most part, the compound word "contact lens" did not exist at that time. There were several options for obtaining visual corrections. Opticians provide corrective lenses and frames. Optometrists are trained in eye care and treatment. Ophthalmologists are medical doctors specializing in eye problems. All three professions are licensed to fit glasses and contacts. For some people, a slightly blurry world was preferable to glasses, if they could manage their daily tasks without problems. To be "good looking" usually meant someone who had attractive physical features without glasses. Movie stars and models of the day usually did not wear glasses in public. One exception was Harold Lloyd, whose glasses were his trademark in comedic silent films and talkies. When children wore glasses at school, they could be teased, ridiculed, and called "four eyes." They were targets for being bullied for looking different. "Bookworm" was a term applied to children with glasses since they tended to be studious and needed to wear their glasses to see. It is no wonder that many avoided wearing . glasses in public unless they needed them. As Dorothy Parker famously said, "Men seldom make passes at girls who wear glasses." One would think there could be a ready market for contact lenses as an invention that could give people perfect vision and a natural look without wearing glasses. There was, with some caveats.

There is a natural fear of putting something in the eye. Most animals have a natural blink reflex when something approaches or gets close to the eye. The eyelid closes to cover and protect the eye from damage whenever something is perceived coming close to the eye. The natural blink reflex must be overcome in order to insert a contact lens into the eye. Contact lens wearers have overcome this problem, but others cannot. A motivating factor helping people overcome their fear is vanity. They think their image in the world is enhanced when they do not have to wear glasses.

There are psychological effects of wearing glasses. For some people, glasses are comforting as a method to distance themselves from other people. This barrier hides who is there. When taken to the extreme, there would be the feeling behind sunglasses that no one would recognize whoever is in this disguise. Mild-mannered Clark Kent, Superman's alter ego, was comfortably hidden behind his black-rimmed glasses and unrecognizable as the Man of Steel. We wear smaller thin-framed light eyeglasses when we wish to be more visible, less ostentatious, studious, and outgoing. Movie stars and fashionistas favor oversized glasses with bold frames. They needed to impress and be fashion leaders, as demonstrated by the cat-eye frames of the 1950s to the oversized colorful Elton John frames. Some professions exclude eyeglasses for various reasons. FAA regulations require 20/20 vision in each eye for pilots. Construction workers and other "manly professions" excluded glasses from a machismo standpoint. Contact sports athletes cannot wear glasses that would shatter and cause safety issues. People in these areas were potential candidates for contact lenses.

Why do people wear contact lenses? From the beginning of widespread acceptance of contact lenses during the 1950s, people primarily wore contact lenses out of vanity. There was freedom to see clearly without being hindered by frames perched on the nose and ears. It allowed us to have a natural appearance and to fit the image of the healthy all-around American who has no impairments. Up until Elton John came on the scene to popularize outrageous eyeglass frames, glasses were a hard sell. Vanity aside, there are real practical and medical reasons for wearing contact lenses.

For sports enthusiasts, there are numerous reasons to choose contact lenses over glasses. There is no concern over breakage of glasses in challenging contact sports such as football, basketball, hockey, or wrestling. When snow or water skiing, there is no restriction from snow or water blurring the glasses. Walking outside from a dry to a humid area, or walking in the rain, there is no fogging of the lenses.

On the practical side of vision, contact lenses offer clear vision without distortions compared to high prescriptions in glasses. There are optical reasons why vision in contacts is better and less distorted than in glasses given a high prescription or prescriptions with large amounts of astigmatism.

Today we have computer-designed cataract lens implants to insert into the eye to replace the eye's internal lens when it becomes cloudy, thus restoring vision. These intraocular cataract lenses are similar to having a contact lens inside the eye rather than on it. In the days before cataract lens implants, thick plus lens glasses were prescribed after surgery. The natural lens in the eye focuses light on the back of the eye. The focusing power of the lens is about +18 diopters. A diopter is a unit of measurement defining the optical power of a lens or mirror. To replace that much focusing power requires a high plus lens, like having a thick magnifying lens. At the time contact lenses developed, they were an excellent solution to the problems patients experienced after cataract surgery. A thin contact lens replaced the old fashioned thick glasses and provided clear distortion-free vision.

When children have crossed eyes (esotropia) or wall-eyes (exotropia), contact lenses can help in the visual correction of these problems. Contacts may be used in conjunction with surgery of the eye muscles, or sometimes in place of that surgical procedure. Babies born with esotropia (crossed eyes) are fitted with plus power contact lenses resulting in correcting both the vision and the strabismus (cross-eyed condition). It is thanks to Dr. Newton K. Wesley that contact lenses became popular. The words "contact lenses" were in the dictionary and popularized after he formed a contact lens manufacturing company in Chicago, Illinois, with his optical partner, Dr. George N. Jessen.

Dr. Wesley fought discrimination and unjust incarceration as a young Japanese American during World War II. His life exemplifies an American drama struggling against systemic racism to fulfil a dream of better vision for himself and others. The company he and his partner formed was eventually called Wesley-Jessen, Inc. Wesley-Jessen was not a company known to the average American until Mitt Romney's run for the 2012 presidential campaign cited Wesley-Jessen. Mitt Romney claimed that he was a businessman with outstanding economic experience through his work as the head of Bain Capital for 15 years. The major success story he touted was Wesley-Jessen, which became a symbol of his successful $6 million investment that became $300 million in four years. Mitt Romney used this as his prize story throughout his campaign. Romney's team ran the commercial on national television news during the campaign. A sign of successful market penetration was symbolized by the news item being satirized on the Daily Show by Jon Stewart.

Wesley-Jessen, Inc. was founded as The Plastic Contact Lens Company (PCL) in 1946. PCL manufactured and sold hard or rigid contact lenses to licensed opticians, optometrists, and ophthalmologists. Because the company sold products to eye care professionals, the identity of the company was not generally known to the public. Dr. Wesley founded the National Eye Research Foundation (NERF) as an educational organization that would instruct doctors on the latest developments in contact lens research and fitting techniques through regional and national meetings. There was also a consumer educational component to inform the public of new developments in the contact lens field.

During the 1950s, the company's sales of contact lenses doubled every month. This rapid expansion put enormous pressure on the production line and management to keep up with the demand. By 1973, Wesley-Jessen had become the most significant contact lens manufacturer in the United States. In 1986 the company had sales of $43 million, and this increased to $95 million by 1986. This book looks at the man behind the development of the idea that contact lenses could be used to save vision. He turned that concept into a reality that helped millions of people to have a quality of life undreamed of in previous centuries. In brief, this biography of Dr. Wesley describes essential accomplishments of his roles in the development of contact lenses in the United States and globally from the 1940s through 1980.

In the 1940s he realized that there was a possible cure for his eye disease, keratoconus. The solution was the development of contact lenses that could be worn more comfortably than the large shells available at the time. He and George Jessen experimented with plastics to develop smaller wearable contact lenses. They and their colleagues created manufacturing procedures to make the new lenses reproducibly to precision standards.

The small novel lenses inserted on the eyes required that doctors be trained in the techniques of making measurements of patients' vision requirements. The measurements are different from those needed for fitting spectacles. Dr. Wesley taught thousands of doctors to fit the lenses, thereby creating specialty practices and a better standard of living. Dr. Wesley was a natural and gifted educator from the earliest days of his optometric career at North Pacific College of Optometry.

Dr. Wesley recognized that the public needed education in the concept and use of wearing contact lenses to overcome the natural fear of placing something on the eye. He fitted movie stars, athletes, politicians, and others with contact lenses, and they helped to create public awareness. Dr. Wesley created the NERF in 1955 to do research and to educate both doctors and the public in new developments in contact lenses.

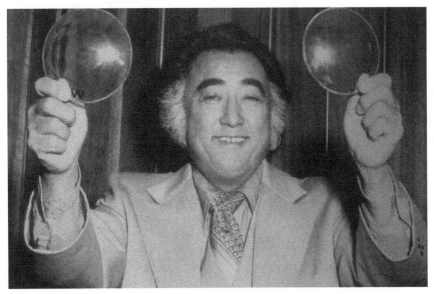

Newton Wesley with demonstration contact lenses, c. 1970. (Roy Wesley personal collection)

1 ORIGINS

Newton Wesley was a Japanese American born Newton Uyesugi to immigrant parents in Westport, Oregon, on October 1, 1917. His family's name, Uyesugi, was challenging for Americans to hear, spell, and remember. How Newton Uyesugi became Newton Wesley is part of the enigma constituting his personality and development, which will unfold in the story of his life and drive to create contact lenses. Newton's father was a laborer in the Westport Lumber Company with hundreds of Japanese immigrant workers. World and local events at the time of birth affected the family's immediate and future lifestyle. The Russian Revolution began in March 1917, and the United States entered World War I during April. Two events reshaped Russia in 1917: the overthrow of the Russian Imperial Romanov family in February of 1917, and then in October, seizure of power by Lenin and the Bolsheviks. These events had global political and social impacts. Westport Lumber joined the US war effort in supplying lumber, especially Sitka Spruce, which was necessary as the supple wood needed for aircraft production. No formal food rationing existed during World War I for the US, but a reduction in food consumption was encouraged so that troops and allies could be fed during the war. There were "Meatless Tuesdays" and "Wheatless Wednesdays." During these austere days of hard labor and stringency, Newton's parents and he himself would never imagine that he was destined to revolutionize the eye care industry in the US and around the globe. Remarkably, a child born to immigrant parents from Japan in a rough lumber camp in Oregon forests could accomplish that.

Five months after Newton's delivery, the 1918 influenza pandemic arrived in the United States with a high mortality rate among infants under five years of age. The family was spared from contagion being in a relatively isolated lumber camp. Newton was born into a time of global change, and he was fated to play a role.

Newton's father, Kojiro Uyesugi, was known as "Harry" in the

US. Kojiro was born into generations of rice farmers in Wakayama Prefecture, Japan, on April 8, 1880. He was the 4th of 9 children. Lured by tales of gold-paved streets and good salaries, thousands of immigrants came from Wakayama. Three thousand seven hundred fifty young Wakayama men emigrated over the years. An area called Little America developed because so many of the young sons went to the United States. Immigrant Japanese labor was needed to work on the railroads, fisheries, farms, and lumber mills in the United States. Kojiro ended up working in all of those industries during his lifetime.

Kojiro emigrated from Japan to the Americas in 1899 at the age of 19 during difficult economic times in Japan. The income from rice farming was insufficient to sustain the family during difficult economic times in the Meiji era. Kojiro arrived legally in the US through British Columbia. Newton's sister, Alice, related that their father made the trip to the US working as a cabin boy on a ship. Upon landing, he worked in the salmon fishery industry, like many young men from Wakayama. Later, Kojiro obtained a job working on a farm. One day he said to his boss, "Hence broke, bacon ran away!" His boss was bewildered. Kojiro was trying to say, "Fence broken, the pig ran away!" Kojiro had a high school education in Japan. Determined to integrate into American ways, he learned English on his own without formal training. Improving English skills became a life-long pursuit for him and his future wife.

Kojiro's older brother, Seikichi, entered the United States illegally, "crawling on his belly," according to his daughter, from Mexico to El Paso, Texas. He first worked in the oil fields of Mexico and then in Texas. He traveled north to Portland to meet up with his younger brother. In 1912, Kojiro began work at the Westport Lumber Company in Oregon. His younger sister was married to Shiogo Shiozaki, the foreman of the company. His brother-in-law was in charge of hiring Japanese workers brought in from Japan and helped Kojiro get a job. Over 250 Japanese immigrants worked at the Westport camp pulling logs from the water, trimming them, sawing them into boards, and resawing them into lumber stock.

Kojiro's job was to pull floating logs out of the Columbia River, measure them, and send them to the mill for cutting. Kojiro worked two of the three shifts, starting in the morning. He rested in the afternoon and returned for the night shift. Hard labor had been a

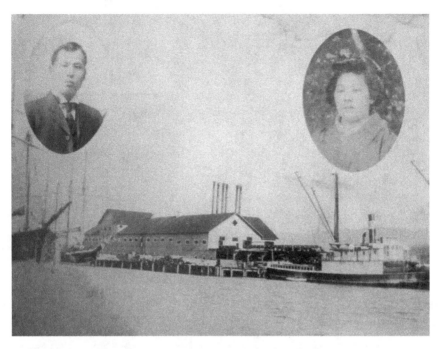

Westport Sawmill and Lumber Company, Westport, Oregon. c. 1900. Left portrait: *Shiogo Shiozaki (Newton's uncle by marriage).* Right portrait: *Suye Uyesugi Shiozaki. Suye was Newton's aunt, Kojiro Uyesugi's sister. (Roy Wesley personal collection)*

fact of life for him as a young man harvesting rice in Japan. He and his brothers loaded the harvest of heavy bags onto a flatbed boat. They sold the rice downriver in Gobo City and then had to pole the boat against the current while walking on the shoreline to get back home. He developed a strong body doing that. He was a muscular, stocky man with a straight military back all his life. Late in life, he was doing sit-ups every morning just after getting up.

Kojiro saved enough money at the lumber mill to return to his village in Japan to marry Chiyo Hata through a baishakunin, a marriage go-between, on December 6, 1914. His bride was 17 years younger than he was. He and his bride returned to the US through Seattle in April 1915.

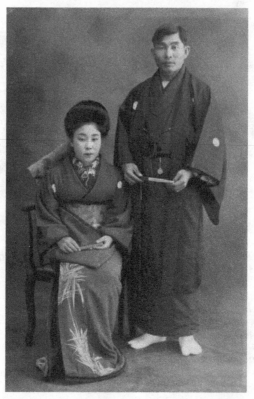

Chiyo Hata and Kojiro Uyesugi wedding portrait, Gobo, Wakayama Prefecture, Japan. December 6, 1914. (Roy Wesley personal collection)

They settled down in the lumber company's village of worker cabins along the Columbia River in Westport, Oregon. The Uyesugi family name means "over the cedar trees." Newton's cousin in Japan, Fumiko Uyesugi, was an energetic 84 years old in 2007 when she guided the Wesley family on a trip to the ancestral home town, Gobo City, in Wakayama Prefecture. She led the way through the narrow village streets to the traditional Japanese house that replaced the original family home where Newton's father and relatives were born. True to the Uyesugi family name, the house sat high over fragrant Japanese cedar trees on a cliff overlooking the Hidaka river and the rice paddies below. Wakayama's resemblance to Westport, Oregon, with its forests of Douglas fir trees and the Columbia River, was striking. The only missing feature was the rice fields.

Newton was the second child of Kojiro and Chiyo Uyesugi. Their first son, Kanji, was born on October 1, 1916. This child tragically died in infancy at the age of three months. Newton was born on October 1, 1917, a year to the day after Kanji's birth. Three children followed: Corinne (1919), Alice (1921), and Edward (1922). The eldest son inherited the privileges and responsibilities of being Ichi-ban, the number one son in a Japanese family. He received favored treatment and status but had to be a model for his siblings as well as watching out and caring for them. Responsibility and duty became traits that lasted throughout his life. His upbringing and early history shaped his personality and character.

Lee and Roy Wesley (Newton's sons) made a trip to Westport, Oregon, in 1960 with Kojiro and Chiyo Uyesugi. They visited the places where the family lived and worked during Newton's childhood. They visited the simple gray granite slab marking the grave of the firstborn Uyesugi son, Kanji, who died in infancy. The grave marker was next to a cherry tree that Kojiro and Chiyo had planted in honor of their baby. Kojiro spoke softly and tenderly, "See, Kanji, here come your nephews Lee and Roy to visit you."

His voice was tinged with emotion that traversed past decades and brought to life the tragedy that had occurred. Years later, when Newton was setting up his first optometric practice in Portland, he added the middle initial "K" in honor of his deceased older brother. People often asked Newton, "What does the initial "K" stand for?" He would reply, "K is just a letter, no name. Newton said, "When I came along, my parents were superstitious and were afraid to name me after the death of their firstborn son, Kanji. They asked the attending physician to name me, and he named me after Sir Isaac Newton."

As Newton grew up, the forests and the broad river of Westport became his playground and a training arena for survival and adventures with his many cousins. They learned to swim, hunt, fish, and explore. The boys grew strong and agile, leaping the floating logs of the lumber mill and swimming to the island in the middle of the river from the campsite. Newton described camping out on the island, eating the fish they caught:

The starry skies and the heavenly jewels sparkling fed the young mind. One could dream and reach for the stars and do anything one would envision. The quiet of the night with the natural sounds of the river, the wind, the trees, and the animals on the island was an environmental blend. Often, during these quiet moments, a deep feeling of loneliness would engulf me while the universe put on a great show for me. (Wesley, autobiography, c. 2005, unpublished manuscript)

He learned to love the beauty of nature and longed to recapture that idyllic time for the rest of his life. Newton missed the forest wilderness when his family moved to the city life of Portland, Oregon. City life was a difficult adjustment for this country boy. He turned inward and experienced a period of shyness, which led to his love of learning and reading books for comfort. He became a voracious reader, taking out several books at a time from the local library. During summer breaks, he returned to Westport to play with his cousins. Hunting and fishing required cunning and cooperation with his cousins and friends. The skills Newton learned in nature's testing grounds were applied to his later business practices when he needed help getting projects started and having others manage tasks to completion.

By 1920, Kojiro saved enough money to buy a farm 90 miles south of Westport, Oregon. The farm had 10 acres of land and a greenhouse where they raised cucumbers. He began his company, Uyesugi and Company. His simple business card on 3 ½" X 2" white paper stock read:

UYESUGI & CO., - GROW ALL KIND OF - OPEN AIR AND GREENHOUSE STOCK- CUCUMBER, FLOWER AND ALL KIND PLANTS. RT. 1, BOX 110, SHERWOOD, ORE.

Newton still enjoyed playing outdoors as he did in Westport and learned to drive a tractor at an early age, using blocks so his feet could reach the pedals. Kojiro and Chiyo worked hard together on their 10-acre farm with a greenhouse for five years. Newton reported that the new farm had to be cleared of trees to plant crops. The trees had to be cut down one by one, the trunks hauled away, and the stumps needed to be removed. His dad harnessed horses to remove some tree stumps. Dynamite blew up stubborn stumps. It was hard work clearing the farmland and then tilling the soil before planting and finally harvesting crops.

It was during these farming days that Newton went to Tualatin Elementary School and began the practice of judo. Farming and practicing the art of self-defense helped him to develop his body and increase his strength. They farmed the land five years, and when Kojiro's hay fever combined with asthma worsened over the years, farming became impossible for him. Kojiro sold the farm and moved to nearby Portland, Oregon, where he invested in a leasehold on the Garland Hotel at 19th and Bismark in 1925 near the Multnomah Stadium. It was an unfortunate investment for Kojiro as he lost money on the deal. Shortly after that, in 1927, he purchased the Villa House, a rooming/boarding hotel in downtown Portland near the waterfront on Columbia and SW First Street. The Villa House was in a rough area of Portland and home to diverse tenants from Norway, Switzerland, Sweden, Italy, Greece, and Japan as well as a variety of American states. Income from the renters helped to get the family through the Great Depression.

Newton said, "I had a great deal of trouble adapting to the big city and making new friends." The transition from being wild and carefree in the woods at the lumber mill in Westport and on the farm in Sherwood and Tualatin was difficult. Newton's constant book reading took a toll on his eyesight. When he was nine, his grades began to drop, and his teacher noticed that Newton couldn't see the blackboard, so she sent him to see "the oculist, Dr. Brown." Newton reluctantly wore his glasses but knew that he had to to see clearly and to function in the world. He became more myopic over time and had to wear thick glasses as his eyes became progressively worse. His sister Alice was so afflicted with poor eyesight that she had to go to a sight-saving school. Being nearsighted and having a difficult adjustment to city life brought Newton into the world of reading books, which helped to satisfy his inquisitive nature. He wrote, "I enjoyed books. On Saturday mornings, I would go to the library and get five or six books, whatever the limit was, and take them home and read them over the weekend. I would read late into the night, and often, when my mother would tell me that I should stop reading

7

so much, I would use a flashlight and read under the bedcovers."

In spite of his bookish nature, Newton also loved sports, especially basketball, which he could practice "by the hour." He had to wear a cage over his eyeglasses because he had so many broken lenses. Other sports attracted him as well. He wanted to become part of his high school baseball team, but he remembers being so introverted that he couldn't summon the courage to try out for the team. When he finally got the nerve as a senior, the coach said he was too old and should have come out in his freshman year. Newton realized he couldn't have done that then because he had to go to Japanese classes after school when the team was practicing.

There was a brief period when Newton's grades dropped because he needed glasses to see better. His teacher recommended that his family take him to an eye doctor. With new glasses, he returned to getting excellent grades. Newton was such a good student that he was promoted beyond his age level into higher grades.

Kojiro found $55 on the steps of the hotel and, unable to find the owner, he used the money to open a grocery store next door to the Villa House. Kojiro thought that the grocery store would help feed the family through the Depression. Kojiro named the grocery store "Newton's Grocery," which reflected his desire that the store be "American" and fit into the community. In this spirit, all the children had been given American names rather than Japanese names. They even lived outside of Portland's Japan Town, which was to the north. In a letter to his sister, Alice, Newton wrote his memory of the grocery store:

> *I remember the cans were so sparse when we first bought material from Hudson Duncan that we could only have one row and only one high on the shelves. I went to work at Azumano's and learned about the way they displayed and sold in the grocery store, so I remodeled the whole thing—over the objections of Dad. I can't remember now, but I remember moving a lot of shelves and put up the signs like Azumano's. Anyway, it worked, and the grocery store did twice as much business, as I recall. I am sure the daily gross wasn't over $50 a day. But, it kept us eating, I'm sure. Everything helped in those days, as you know.*
> (Wesley, letter dated March 6, 1989)

Newton and Cecilia gave birth to their sons Lee (1940) and Roy (1942) at the Villa House.

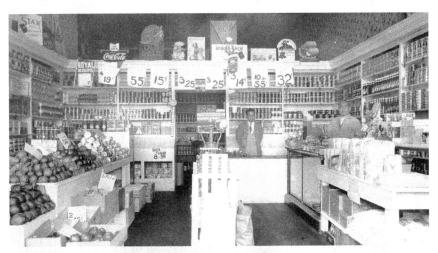

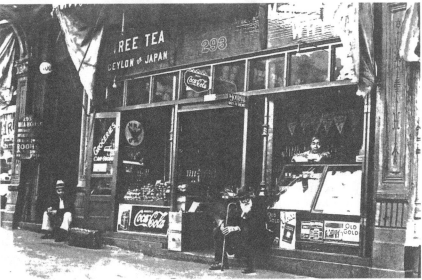

TOP: *"Newton's Grocery" about 1935.* Center: *Vito Rancalli.* Right: *Kojiro "Harry" Uyesugi.* BOTTOM: *Exterior of "Newton's Grocery." To the far left is the entrance to the Villa House. The two seated men were tenants of the hotel. c. 1935. (Roy Wesley Personal collection)*

Newton was a quick learner and graduated from Portland's Lincoln High School when he was 16 years old. He had no idea what he wanted to do. He wished he could continue his education, but realized that he needed time to mature. Being younger because of grade skipping, he was always the smallest in his class. After graduating, he decided to go to Hidden Inlet, Alaska, to work in the salmon cannery. He moved to Astoria, Oregon for one month in August, 1938 to work at the Columbia River Packers Association salmon cannery while living on 6th Street. He did more hard physical labor pulling railroad ties on the Oregon Trunk Line in Western Oregon. Working in the desert pulling railroad ties up and pounding spikes led to a 25-pound loss, resulting in his being a skinny 111 lb after three months. Newton's 1940 draft card listed his height at 5' 10" and weight at 170 pounds. His final hard labor job was found through the aid of his uncle Shiogo Shiozaki, the father of his cousins and playmates growing up at the Westport Lumber camp, which was still there 17 years after his birth at the site. Newton's uncle got him a job to help him raise funds to go to college. Westport Lumber management reduced the workforce to dozens of men from the 250 immigrants working in 1917. Some remaining workers helped train Newton to become a resaw workman (the person who saws the previously cut boards into desired shapes). The lumber camp was the ultimate work experience that forced him to realize that he had to better himself or face a grim future. Newton observed the life of the lumbermen: "The big thing was to go bowling at the 4L, drink beer, go to the island and have a picnic, chase the girls, ride motorcycles, play sports, or do all the sundry things young men of that age did." He wanted something more than that. He remembered that his mother wanted him to become a doctor, but that was not appealing because, as he said, "I did not like the sight of blood." The 4L Hall in Westport was a center for social life. 4L stood for the Loyal Legion of Loggers and Lumberman, a local group preventing unionization by the International Workers of the World.

2 THE ROAD TO NORTH PACIFIC COLLEGE OF OPTOMETRY

Newton had saved enough money to pursue his college dream but had no idea what profession to choose. He sat down with the Portland Yellow Pages, the business telephone book practically nonexistent in today's world. Starting with the "A" listings while looking for an occupation that would interest him, he got to the "O's" and found OPTOMETRY. Somehow that word and all that it implied was for him. Perhaps his childhood experience of needing glasses to see was a compelling factor in the decision. Newton wrote about the experience:

> ...I saw the word optometry. That appealed to me. It had to do with the eyes, one received a doctor's degree, and there was no blood. It fitted all my requirements and I was happy. The same classified ads, under Schools, showed a school of optometry in Portland, Oregon. How lucky could I get? I could go to school and live at home with my family. That appealed to me also, since I wanted to be with them. (Wesley, 1988 pp. 21-22)

He wrote for application forms and applied to North Pacific School of Optometry. Dr. Fording interviewed and accepted him for admission. Optometry, as a profession, was not universally licensed and accredited by academic institutions in 1936 when Newton entered the school. The National Association for the Accreditation of Colleges did not recognize the Doctor of Optometry degree. Degree recognition became a mission for Newton and his colleagues, Clary Carkner and Roy Clunes, after graduating.

The school was founded in January 1921 by Harry Lee Fording, president, OphD., D.O.S. North Pacific occupied a floor in the now historic Selling Building at 610 SW Alder Street (now the Oregon National Building). A letter written by Dr. Fording printed in the *Optical Journal and Review*, May, 1923, stated:

In pursuance of public supervision in the use of optometrical knowledge and skill, there was founded in 1921 a school of optometry and optics, known as the Oregon College of Ocular Sciences, an institute of learning chartered by the State of Oregon and licensed to confer the degree, Doctor of Ocular Sciences. The course embraces not only the study of optometry, but also the study of optics, or the manufacture of lenses and frames, and their adjustment to the eye and face.

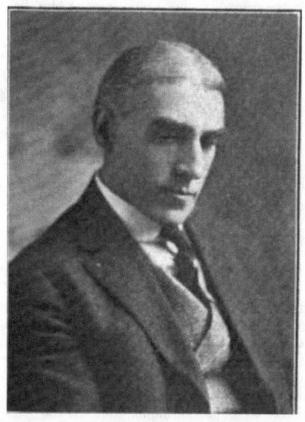

Dr. Harry Lee Fording. (Optical Journal and Review, *May 10, 1923)*

The 1923 *Optical Journal and Review* continued,

> Perhaps Dr. Fording's reputation as a Greek scholar, as a student of law, theology and medicine may explain his insistence on a higher standard of general education as well as in optometry. Hence, in the course of instruction are included mathematics, physics, histology and general anatomy and physiology.

Newton enthusiastically accepted the academic rigors imposed by Dr. Fording when he said that, before attending his first classes, Dr. Fording sent books to study in anatomy, physiology and optics before school started. He read the books with interest and enthusiasm while he worked two shifts to make more money before the start of his first semester.

To raise enough cash while at school, Newton worked at the University Club of Portland at SW 1225 6th Avenue, assisting the chefs, taking care of their knives, and as a dishwasher. It was an easy seven minute walk from his home at the Villa House to the University Club.

In September 1936, a month shy of his 19th birthday, Newton began his much anticipated curriculum at North Pacific College of Optometry. Dr. Fording separated the Optometry College from the North Pacific College of Oregon Schools of Dentistry and Pharmacy. He then moved to another historic 1911 building at 809 NE 6th Avenue across the river. He finally moved the Optometry College to the Hollywood Arcade building on the 2nd floor adjacent to and connected with the Hollywood Theatre at 4112 NE Sandy Boulevard. Newton took optometry classes at this location. He joined eight other students in his first-year class, and they formed part of the 50 total enrollees in the school that year. Newton's father presented him with the gift of a second-hand 1935 Ford to celebrate his admission to the school. He could save time and drive the four miles from his home across the Willamette River to the school in the northeast section of Portland. He reported, "The school was about fifteen minutes away by car from where we lived; the proximity delighted me." Newton buried himself in his studies, as shown by his converting the closet in his small room at the Villa house into his study area where he could concentrate without distractions.

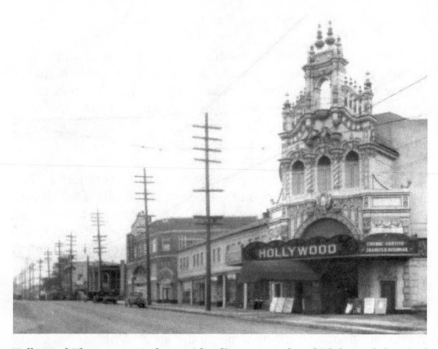

Hollywood Theatre, 1926 photo with adjacent arcade, which housed the North Pacific College of Optometry on the second floor. (Architectural Heritage Center, Portland, Oregon)

In December 1937, the Optometric Associations of Oregon, Washington, and British Columbia, held their annual six-day meeting in Portland's historic Multnomah Hotel (built 1912) from December 11 to the 17th. Newton registered as a student for $2.00 to attend all meetings of the Northwest Congress of Optometry (as the combined meeting was called). The program included over 15 hours of lectures in Analytical Optometry by the noted Arthur Marten Skeffington (1890-1976), the father of behavioral optometry and co-founder of the Optometric Extension Program. Another highlighted speaker was Theodore Alfred Brombach, author of visual fields textbooks and developer of color visual fields. Brombach presented 8 hours of lectures. Newton was influenced theoretically and practically by Skeffington and Brombach. Skeffington impacted Newton's thinking in behavioral and vision therapy, especially when he opened his Chicago eye practice specializing in those areas. Fifty years later, Newton remembered and revived Brombach's concept of color visual fields as a possible way to "empty half the hospitals in the U.S." if color fields were applied early to help diagnose diseases. For example, Brombach demonstrated that smoking decreased red, blue, green visual fields significantly and was detrimental to health. Toward the end of his life, Newton remembered Brombach's theories and invested some of his assets in the development of computerized color vision fields. Dale Agonis, an automation engineer, created the automated system for Newton. The re-introduction of 1930 concepts did not gain wide application or acceptance. Although T.A. Brombach practiced in San Francisco and was a lecturer at the Berkeley School of Optometry, his work was recognized when in 1967, Pacific University's College of Optometry named a new wing of the school for him, illustrating his lasting contributions to the field.

After Newton's first academic year, he impressed Dr. Fording so much that he asked Newton to teach geometric optics to the incoming freshman. Newton was only in his second year. Newton felt unqualified and protested, but Fording wouldn't take no for an answer, so Newton ended up teaching the course. Upon graduating from optometry school, President Fording told Newton that he wanted to retire and offered to give Newton the school without charge. Dr. Fording hoped that the school and his legacy would continue. Newton felt that he had to pay something, and he wanted to start his clinical eye practice. He persuaded his classmate, Roy Clunes, to split a $5,000 purchase fee and run the school with him. Newton was 20 years old, and the country was in the midst of the Great Depression, so coming up with cash was difficult, but both Newton and Roy managed to get a bank loan for the purchase.

At the same time, Newton enlisted another fellow student, Clarence (Clary) Carkner, to join them in running the school. It was Dr. Carkner, who, years later, was instrumental in obtaining academic recognition for PCO as an accredited school of optometry. After the war, North Pacific College of Optometry was merged into Pacific University. It became the Pacific University School of Optometry in 1945. The school's co-owners, Newton and Roy Clunes, negotiated through correspondence with Pacific University during the war years to pave the way for the merger.

Newton never forgot his exciting years which began his career at North Pacific College of Optometry. He maintained lifelong connections with his friends and colleagues, Clary Carkner and Roy Clunes. The three comrades served together as Trustees of the Pacific University College of Optometry for many years during the 1950s. Dr. Wesley was a generous contributor to Pacific College of Optometry.

There was never a time in his life when there was just one thing happening. A multitude of tasks was always at hand. While Newton was in optometry school learning his new profession and teaching, he was involved with the Japanese American community, including the Japanese American Citizens League (JACL). He became the president of the Portland chapter of JACL at the age of twenty-three. Newton played on the basketball team and was active in the church community that traveled between Portland and Seattle for games and social dances. It was during these activities that he met and fell in love with Cecilia K. Sasaki, a beautiful and lively young girl from Seattle. He courted her for three years and, in time, convinced her to get a job and move to Portland from Seattle so that they could deepen their relationship. They were married at the Centenary Methodist Church in Portland, Oregon, by the Reverend Guy Goodsell. It was unusual because the pastor of the Epworth Methodist Church, Reverend Goto, was the minister to his parents and the family. In response to a question about this change, Newton said that he and the Reverend Goto "didn't get along."

There was a hidden backstory to this episode which caused the break between Newton and his family's minister. Roy Wesley reported:

> *I realized that as I grew up, I never saw my parents celebrate their wedding anniversary. I thought that it was because Newton was always busy, traveling, and consumed by the challenges of developing his business. After a couple of years of searching many sites for marriage certificates, I wrote to the Portland Marriage License Section with different dates to obtain a copy of their marriage license. You have to provide a specific date for them to retrieve a marriage license. I found the date of their marriage: June 9, 1940, with Rev. Goodsell as the officiant. I finally had a date to put on the wedding photo that I have on their*

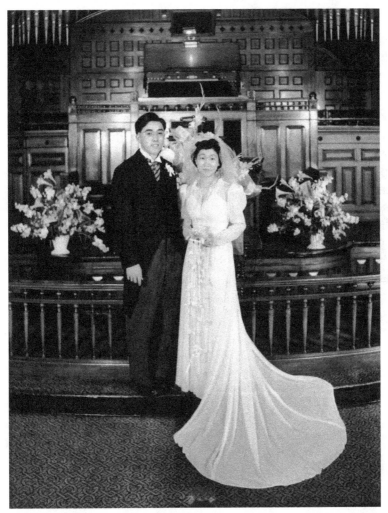

Newton Uyesugi (Wesley) and Cecilia Sasaki wedding at Centenary Methodist Church, Portland, Oregon, June 9, 1940. (Roy Wesley personal collection)

wedding day in front of the altar. Mom looks frail and wan in the demurely elegant white wedding dress with a modest train made by her mother. Her mother probably noticed the slight tummy bump since she made her wedding gown and did the fittings for the dress. She must have realized the truth of what had happened. News like that could not be hidden in a tightly knit Japanese community. It may have caused consternation and a rift between Newton and the Reverent Goto at the Epworth Japanese Methodist Church. Nonetheless, to all outward appearances, everything was proper. It was a traditional wedding with Newton, his best man, and the wedding party in formal black wedding coats with tails. (Roy Wesley, personal recollection)

Newton and Cecilia celebrated the birth of their first son Newton Lee Uyesugi on December 9, 1940. To avoid any confusion of having two Newtons in the family, they called him by his middle name, Lee, rather than his first name. The traditional Japanese *Hatsuzekku* (first celebration of life) was celebrated to ensure this firstborn child's growth and to protect him against bad luck in the future. A display of Japanese dolls included a samurai on a white horse. On a separate wooden stand was placed an ornate *kabuto*, the traditional samurai helmet.

3 WORLD WAR II

On a clear, crisp, quiet Sunday morning in Portland, December 7, 1941, Newton was leaving his night watch duty at the reception desk of one of his father's hotels in a poor section of town. He was driving home to the Villa House about 11:30 am in the 1935 secondhand Ford he received as a graduation gift from his parents when he heard on the car radio,

> *We have witnessed this morning from a distance, a view of a brief full battle of Pearl Harbor and a severe bombing of Pearl Harbor by enemy planes, undoubtedly Japanese. The city of Honolulu has also been attacked, and considerable damage done. This battle has been going on for nearly three hours. One of the bombs dropped within fifty feet of KGU tower. It is no joke, it is a real war.* (WABC News, 1941-12-07, Library of Congress, 2001664035)

NBC broadcast the news just minutes after the beginning of the attack when the station received a telephone call from a Honolulu reporter giving details of planes flying overhead and bombing. Later that afternoon, Newton picked up special editions of *The Oregonian* and the *Oregon Journal*. The papers described the chaos of the day. They reported many rumors, including one that a Japanese pilot was shot down and was wearing an Oregon State ring. Most of these were later proven to be false. Newton knew Marshall Dana the publisher, and editor of the *Oregon Journal*, and Palmer Hoyt, the publisher of *The Oregonian*. The papers interviewed him because he was the president of the Portland Japanese American Citizens League (JACL). His main task was to talk about the loyalty of the Japanese American community to the United States. His comments fell on deaf ears in a city frozen in terror.

Japanese Americans changed from being racially invisible in the white population to becoming visible targets for discrimination and racial epithets. Vigilante patriots roamed the streets targeting Asian faces with tomatoes and racial insults.

Oregon's Governor Charles Sprague immediately ordered police across the state "to be vigilant and guard essential structures and services and hold enemy aliens under surveillance." Portland's Mayor Earl Riley directed that brigades guard critical areas in the city, and the police chief mobilized the officers and 200 reserve officers. Newton was one of the reserve officers. He was a member of the Portland auxiliary fire department and the police department. Newton worked with the Portland police guarding bridges and other potential targets at night. He also worked with the FBI, answering questions they had about the Japanese immigrants he knew to determine loyalties. The Western Command and Fourth Army set up curfews for Japanese Americans to be off the streets between 8 pm to 6 am. Newton was amazingly exempt because of his auxiliary police and fire status and his work with the FBI.

Meanwhile, Newton's good friend, Min Yasui, wanted to test the constitutionality of the curfew by being arrested in violation of the ruling. When no one stopped him on the street, he walked into a police station, and the police had to put him under arrest. Newton said, "He and I would have many discussions on the violation of the Constitutional rights of Japanese-Americans (Nisei) prior to evacuation."

Newton was only 24 years old at the time, but already connected to political figures in the city and state. Newton wrote, "I was very involved in community affairs and in the Japanese-American communities, also. Through the college, I was involved with the governor because of regulations relating to the College of Optometry as well as the state board members, and I would meet with Governor Sprague of Oregon from time to time." It is unknown how he managed to work along with his fellow Caucasian firefighters and police during this period of anti-Japanese hysteria. Somehow he was accepted by those who were designated protectors of the city.

In January 1942, Newton and other community leaders appealed to the Portland City Council not to rescind the business licenses of the first-generation Japanese. On January 28, 1942, the City Council ignored their arguments and unanimously revoked all business licenses of Issei (first-generation Japanese). In addition, the personnel board stopped civil service employment to "citizens of German, Italian or Japanese blood. Three weeks later, the state fired thirteen Nisei civil service workers and seven board of equalization employees."

Crude articles and posters appeared, describing and illustrating how to tell the Japanese from Chinese. The stereotypes were inaccurate, insensitive, and offensive. The otherwise lovable children's cartoonist Theodore Geisel, "Dr. Seuss," drew anti-Japanese cartoons before and during World War II. A widely circulated cartoon titled "Waiting for the signal from home" showed lines of same-faced Japanese Americans along the Pacific Coast waiting to pick up TNT packages from a building with the sign "Honorable 5th Column." (The term "fifth column" originated in 1936 during the Spanish Civil War, meaning a group of people who undermine from within to favor the enemy.) The cartoon depicted Japanese Americans as untrustworthy and unpatriotic.

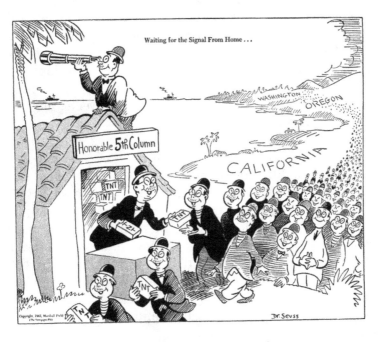

Dr. Seuss, "Waiting for the Signal from Home." PM, *February 13, 1942. (UC San Diego Special Collections)*

Amidst the anti-Japanese hysteria, Newton and his family were spared from the first series of roundups of prominent Japanese American families. Newton assisted the FBI in their search for suspect aliens to detain and through the fortuitous befriending of the captain of the FBI search team, Mr. Grossenbacher. Newton's recollection of this period reveals a human wartime story:

I remember also during this period being awakened by the FBI, being taken around the city of Portland, and being asked various questions about the families who lived in the homes or businesses where I was taken. Later on, I realized that every one of these people were taken into custody and exchanged on the Gripsholm. The Gripsholm was the Swedish ship on which about three thousand Japanese aliens were exchanged for prisoners of war taken by the Japanese. The United States didn't have anyone to exchange on the American side, so we exchanged Japanese nationals who lived in the United States — our parents. I presume all the spies and people who were involved in ambassadorial work had already returned to Japan....during World War II, we captured very few Japanese prisoners. The Japanese prisoners of war would kill themselves before surrendering. Hence, the exchange was arranged between the two governments through Sweden.

We theorized about whether our phones were tapped; we had a suspicion but weren't sure. Often we would lay plans and the FBI would know of our plans, so we felt that they did know. For instance, under the curfew we weren't supposed to be out and we would name a certain place for a meeting. We would see the FBI men, whom we knew, cruising and watching. Perhaps they had other reasons for doing what they did and they found out through other means, but we thought that our phones were tapped. There was one instance that showed me, at least, that we knew of the impending period way beforehand and that we weren't exactly asleep as Americans.

As I was closing my office and my father was helping me pack the various pieces of furniture and equipment, a Mr. Grossenbacher came in to see me and to say "Good-bye."

He said that he was very sorry that I had to leave and that he didn't question my loyalty. I remembered him as a kindly printer whose daughter I had helped. He had come into my office and stated that he was a printer in a nearby shop and that his daughter had poor eyes, and he wanted me to examine her eyes. I did the examination and supplied the prescription without charge — I felt he was as poor as I! In the year or two that passed, he would often come in and talk to me about my philosophies, and we would have long chats between patients. My father seemed very excited when Mr. Grossenbacher left, and I said, "Dad, let's talk later."

At dinnertime he explained to me that Mr. Grossenbacher was the so-called captain or leader of the FBI team that searched the house and then when they turned to the leader and asked, "Are we taking this man in?" the captain said, "No." They asked, "Did you find anything?" And he said, "No." They had found nothing of interest in the search through the house. (Wesley, 1988, pp. 38-39)

Formerly neutral citizens looked at Newton and other Japanese Americans suspiciously at first sight. This behavior made daily life on the streets of Portland uncomfortable and provoked anxiety with Pearl Harbor on everyone's mind. A clear distinction between the real enemies in Japan and loyal Japanese American citizens was not made. Since Japanese Americans looked like the enemy, they were regarded and treated as if they were the enemy.

Newton testified at the Tolan Committee Hearings in Portland on March 12, 1942. Congressman John Tolan entered Congress in 1935 as a New Deal liberal. His committee began in 1940 as the Select Committee to Investigate the Interstate Migration of Destitute Citizens. The issue was the displacement of refugees from the Dust Bowl moving to the West. In 1942, the committee considered testimonies for or against the mass removal of Japanese Americans from the West Coast. The Committee took statements from both sides in Los Angeles, San Francisco, and Portland. Here is a portion of the transcript:

The committee met at 2 p. m. in the United States circuit court room, in the United States Court House, Portland, Oreg., pursuant to notice, Hon. John H. Tolan (chairman) presiding.

Present were: Representatives John H. Tolan (chairman), of California; John J. Sparkman, of Alabama; and Laurence J. Arnold, of Illinois.

TESTIMONY OF HITO OKADA, NATIONAL TREASURER JAPANESE-AMERICAN CITIZENS LEAGUE; DR. NEWTON UYESUGI, PRESIDENT, PORTLAND CHAPTER, JAPANESE-AMERICAN CITIZENS LEAGUE; MAMARO WAKASUGI, JAPANESE-AMERICAN GROWER, OF BANKS, OREG.

Mr. Arnold. You gentlemen will have to pronounce your names for the reporter and spell them, perhaps, and tell what you represent and where you live.

Mr. Uyesugi. My name is Newton Uyesugi. I am president of the Portland Chapter of the Japanese-American Citizens League.

Mr. Arnold. Mr. Uyesugi, how many Japanese aliens and American citizens are there in the State of Oregon?

Mr. Uyesugi. Around 4,071; that is taken from the Oregon Voter.

Mr. Arnold. Do you have these figures for the city of Portland?

Mr. Uyesugi. Yes. Citizens, 955; aliens, 725.

Mr. Arnold. Not quite half, then, of the Japanese within the State are within Portland? There are 1,680 out of 4,071 here in Portland?

Mr. Uyesugi. That is right.

Mr. Arnold. We would like to have you give us a brief description of the Japanese community here in Portland.

Mr. Uyesugi. Well, as was said, there are approximately 1,600 Japanese and Japanese-American citizens in the city of Portland.

I presume the average age of the alien Japanese is about 65; the citizens are about 18 to 20. Their type of business is mostly hotels and apartments, barber shops, laundries, cleaners and dyers, grocery stores, and fruit stands. That will probably take in the majority. I have some figures here. I don't know just exactly what you wanted, but I will be glad to give you these figures. I have had them compiled for you.

The Chairman. You can leave them with the reporter.

(United States Congress. House of Representatives. Select Committee Investigating National Defense Migration. 77th Congress, 2nd sess. *National Defense Migration* (Tolan Committee hearings), Part 30, p. 11433)

Although Newton hoped to influence the committee to give justice to the Japanese Americans in Portland and the State of Oregon, there was not a formal opportunity to do so. The implications of his testimony were the statistic that 57% of Japanese Americans living in Portland were American citizens and should not be deprived of their rights. The citing of the numerous business that these citizens were providing would be lost to the community and their lives disrupted.

The majority of those testifying argued for the removal of Japanese Americans, especially politicians, business owners, and citizens. The issue was whether anyone of Japanese descent could be a loyal American citizen. A minority of voices argued otherwise and were against blatant racism. Newton had a personal relationship with Portland's mayor, Earl Riley. The mayor supported Newton immediately after Pearl Harbor by writing letters on his behalf to release him from the incarceration camp. These actions did not compel the mayor to vote against the mass evacuation. Only the mayors of Berkeley, California, and Tacoma, Washington, supported the rights of the Japanese Americans. As a result, the Tolan Commission did not stand against mass removal.

Involuntary Loss of Home and Work

Executive order 9066, signed by President Roosevelt on February 19,

1942, created chaos for Newton, his family, and 120,000 Japanese Americans. The order removed Americans of Japanese decent from the West Coast to interior military controlled incarceration camps for "protection against espionage and against sabotage to national-defense material...." As a result, he had to close his optometric practice, suspend operations of North Pacific College of Optometry, and settle the hotel properties owned and leased by his father. Newton wrote about this turbulent time:

> Since there were so many hotels being sold at the same time and I knew that I couldn't get a fair price for the hotel my father owned, I went to his partners and asked them to set up absentee management. They stated that this was not possible, we could lose everything, and it was better to get whatever we could for the leasehold, which had four years to run. I tried to have them see it my way, but again fear of not knowing what the future would bring drove them to decide to get rid of everything they could. I finally left it on the basis that I didn't want to sell my shares, but they could sell theirs and I would match the price they could get. It was all right with them. They kept insisting that they would be able to sell it and they had a buyer.
>
> It turned out that the buyer kept lowering his price as the evacuation day approached (May 5, 1942), and they soon learned that no one wanted to pay a fair price.... They would get very little out of their holdings. I did match the original offer price and bought their shares out but, in the interim, I thought it was better, since one of the partners was my father's younger brother, that he should try to the last minute, otherwise he might think I had robbed him if it worked out for the better. At the end, he was begging and insisting almost to the point of becoming violent that I buy his shares, which I finally did at my original offer. It turned out that by keeping management in place I was able to net about ten thousand dollars a year for three years and all their fears did not occur. That's how I managed to bridge the financial gap between the evacuation and the time that it took to relocate. (Wesley, 1988, pp. 36-37)

4 PERSONAL FREEDOM PLANS

Newton was a planner who tackled life crises head-on. He was a doer who took problems or difficult jobs one after the other. He sought solutions when other people succumbed to the circumstances and floundered. During the wartime crisis, he used his political connections to stay free from incarceration and explored all possible avenues to secure his right to live in freedom.

The Quakers, the Society of Friends, were a religious group that supported pacifism and equality for all. Among the many causes actively supported by the Quakers were the abolition of slavery, gender equality for women, prison reform, and refuge for the Japanese Americans placed in the internment camps. Quaker assistance for Japanese Americans stands out as an example of principled courage against the raging current of hate and prejudice that faced the nation at the time. Earlham was founded as a Quaker school. The president of Earlham at the time was William Cullen Dennis, who served as president from 1929 to 1946. Before Newton's arrival in the fall semester in 1942, Dennis accepted two Japanese American transfer students from Whittier College. He thought that up to a dozen more qualified students might be taken in. These transfers were a precedent that helped pave the way for Newton, his brother, and others to be accepted for admission.

After many negotiations with the War Relocation Authority, various universities, and other groups, permission was granted to Earlham and about 600 different colleges in the United States to accept a limited number of Japanese American students for continued education during the war. Approximately 4,000 students were kept out of the incarceration camps to further their education during the war years. To gain admittance, Newton was able to secure letters of recommendation and support about his character and loyalty to the United States as a citizen from prominent people and friends, including:

- Charles A. Sprague, Governor of the State of Oregon
- Earl Riley, Mayor of Portland
- Ralph C. Clyde, Commissioner of Public Utilities, City of Portland
- Dr. Harry Lee Fording, President of North Pacific College of Optometry
- Kermit Wilson, newspaper reporter, and close friend
- Palmer Hoyt, Publisher of *The Oregonian*
- E.B. McNaughton, President, The First National Bank of Portland, Oregon
- J.W. Reed, Methodist Minister, Portland
- Roy B. Clunes, OD, President of North Pacific College of Optometry, Classmate, and friend

On April 21, 1942, Newton wrote a letter on his business stationery to President William Dennis at Earlham College in Richmond, Indiana, requesting admission as a student two weeks before imprisonment:

> *At the present time I am a practicing optometrist; and I am also teaching four classes at the college.*
>
> *Because I am president of the Portland Chapter of the Japanese American Citizens League my work has kept me so busy I have not had the opportunity to apply for admission to your university before this time. I would like to continue my school if it is at all possible and the military authorities will allow me to do so. ...*
>
> *I am married and have a son. At the present time I am only making an application for myself to leave this area and enter school. My family will remain in the resettlement area until conditions are more favorable.*
> (Uyesugi, Letter to President Willam Dennis, 1942)

Was he realistic about the assessment to continue his education? There were no precedents for this situation, and there were no precedents for education exemptions. He did not mention that his wife was pregnant with their second child and in the final month before delivery. Newton's second son was about to be born just 14 days after he wrote this letter. A twist of fate timed the baby's birth on the very day of the family's evacuation order, May 5, 1942. The second child's birth was not as auspicious as that of his first son, Lee. Still, the delivery did temporarily delay the imprisonment deadline. Newton named the child Roy after his schoolmate, Dr. Roy Clunes, and for his good friend and newspaper reporter, Kermit Wilson. Newton described the birth of Roy Kermit Uyesugi (Wesley):

> Roy was born at 5:00 am at home without a doctor (our family doctor, Robert Shiomi, was already an inmate of the camp). Even though I was there, I had to admit he was a self-delivery. Roy Kermit kicked himself to freedom! (Wesley, 1988, p. 40)

It was probably a combination of panic and fear that coursed through the body of Roy's mother, resulting in a premature arrival of a five-pound, nine-ounce boy. The family lost routine and orderliness in the chaos of the times. Familiar things inside their home were gone, and only bare essentials remained. There was no comfort left as she went into labor. She must have wondered, "Into what kind of world am I delivering my child?" Roy was born at home in the Villa House hotel at 5 am, and mother and child went to the Good Samaritan Hospital immediately after delivery. The War Relocation Authority allowed them three days in the hospital to recover from childbirth.

On the war front, unbelievable carnage was occurring as soldiers were shooting, throwing grenades, and being subjected to attacks. Savage gunfire and rocket attacks surrounded them. War raged on multiple European fronts in Germany, Poland, Czechoslovakia, France, the Netherlands, Belgium, Norway, Denmark, Italy, and North Africa. Fierce fighting was simultaneously going on throughout Southeast Asia in Japan, Burma, China, Thailand, Indochina, Malaysia, and the Philippines. Newsreels in the movie theaters, radio reports, and the newspapers described or showed the atrocities of war for the 3½ years the United States was involved. A national draft was instituted in September 1940 before the US entered the war effort in December.

Prison

On May 8, 1942, Cecilia and her son, Roy, were transported from Portland's Good Samaritan Hospital to the grounds of the Pacific International Livestock and Exposition Center in North Portland adjacent to the Columbia River. Newton and son Lee were already imprisoned at the stockyards on May 5, as required by law. The family would live in the hastily modified livestock pens for five months while the Minidoka campsite was being prepared in the south central desert of Idaho. Newton and his family shared a twelve by twelve foot area raw plywood pen with his parents. Wood planks covered the dirt floors where animals were penned. Animal manure was embedded in the soil, resulting in a persistent pungent odor. Flies bred in the fertile manure and infested all the living quarters and the mess hall during meals. The government's solution was to hand out sticky yellow flypaper, which hung from every quarter. Rats and their attendant lice were other hazards, leading to traps and periodic fumigations. Cecilia harbored fears and anxieties as she adjusted to this sordid life. If there were a positive side to living in a germ-infested environment, it would be that the family was exposed to enough bacteria to activate their immune systems. Some natural immunity against pathogens could be a result. Wire fences with barbed wire surrounded the hastily constructed living quarters with armed guards at every corner. More than 3,500 souls lived under these conditions for five to six months until they were shipped by train to the desert incarceration camp at Minidoka, Idaho.

In contrast to the daily reality of their harsh life, Newton's "Letters to Freedom" to the outside world were upbeat. These letters were written and typed by his administrative secretary while he was in confinement, as part of the five-man administration of the detention camp. Some were sent to Governor Sprague and are in the Oregon State Archives. He demonstrated that Japanese Americans were loyal American citizens who could make the best of any situation. Newton gave a positive spin to their plight:

> *On the whole, everyone is taking the situation very nicely. We are doing our utmost to keep up the morale of the people. I must say there is not one of us who would rather*

not be outside of these walls since this is so abnormal. Having a great number of people cooped up together in one place is not exactly to anyone's liking; but the general attitude is that since we must stay here, we will make the best of it. Everyone agrees that since he has been put into the center, he has received every consideration and fair treatment. (Uyesugi, Letter to Governor Sprague, 1942)

Once Newton was in the Portland Assembly Center, some inmates thought he let them down and considered him a traitor because, as JACL President, he worked with the city government. They felt he didn't do enough to keep them free despite his testimonies to the City Council and Tolan Commission. There was resentment about his aiding and abetting the FBI. Nonetheless, he was selected to be part of a five-person administrative council under the civilian administrator, Mr. Emil Sandquist, and his assistant Mr. Booker. Newton volunteered to provide examinations and prescriptions to the inmates. He was allowed to bring his optometric equipment to do eye examinations and supply glasses at cost. No one could profit while in detention.

Newton thought he could serve his country better as a free citizen. In that spirit, he made personal appeals to people who might help him keep his freedom. He called Oregon Governor Charles A. Sprague, Portland's Mayor Earl Riley, City Commissioners Ralph Clyde, and Kenneth Cooper. Newton wrote concerning his contacts that "...they said they would do all they possibly could." Newton added,

I couldn't see being put behind barbed wire for something I didn't do, and I was going to try everything possible to get out. I had served the city of Portland for many years and had never asked for a favor. They were grateful to me and felt that the whole matter wasn't right, and they asked me to do a great deal of paperwork, such as getting letters of recommendation, my history, etc., which I did for a period of two months while I was in the camp.
(Wesley, 1988, pp. 39-40)

Newton's younger brother, Edward Uyesugi, wrote letters to President Roosevelt and members of Congress. He requested that he be permitted to continue his education at a university to be of service to the country. Ed Uyesugi discontinued his education at Willamette College (Salem, Oregon). They received positive responses from Cornell and Earlham College.

As a result of his community work and political connections, Newton received many letters of support, which granted him an early release from incarceration at the Portland Assembly Center. These letters of recommendation were part of the file that the National Japanese American Student Relocation Council (NJASRC) processed for Newton and Edward. It was thanks to the heroic efforts of the many Quakers involved in the NJASRC that so many Japanese American students were able to be freed from unjust imprisonment. According to the *Densho Encyclopedia*:

> The National Japanese American Student Relocation Council (NJASRC) worked during World War II to help resettle inmates from the government's concentration camps to colleges in the Midwest and the East Coast. Under the sponsorship of the American Friends Service Committee (AFSC), the Council worked with students, their families, and the larger Japanese American community as well as a wide range of public and private organizations in ultimately helping more than 4,000 students resettle to pursue their higher education at more than 600 institutions. (Austin, "National Japanese American Student Relocation Council")

The NJASRC worked tirelessly under hostile circumstances to place students. Their humanitarian role and the team of dedicated workers has been largely ignored in history. A NJASRC organization chart showed the extensive network headed by an Executive Committee at the Friends Philadelphia office under Dr. Robert Sproul as chairman. Under the committee were three divisions in Southern California, Northern California, and the Pacific Northwest. These were staffed by many people to distribute information, accept and process applications, and to coordinate placements (National Student Relocation Council, 1942). Newton and his brother, Ed, went to Earlham College in Indiana for further education under the protection and auspices of the Quakers, who were pacifists and opposed the unjust treatment of the Japanese Americans. Nineteen forty-two and the preceding year were stressful for Newton, who was working at many projects simultaneously for long hours every day. He had been getting only 3 to 4 hours of sleep a night. Excessive demands caused his vision to deteriorate rapidly to the point that he saw hundreds of images that would not go away. When Newton looked at a single tree, there would be up to 100 images of that tree in each eye. Trying to read text was a frustrating task in deciphering the jungle of duplicated letters and words that overlapped and created visual and mental chaos. At the time, there was no cure, and no prescription for glasses could correct the defect.

5 EARLHAM COLLEGE

After three months (May–July 1942) in detention at the Portland Assembly Center, Newton left during August 1942. He reported later that it was a difficult decision to leave his incarcerated family. Still, he was determined "not to rot in camp," and after discussing the matter with his family, he decided to take advantage of the opportunity. His firstborn son, Lee, had become ill because of the unsanitary conditions in the stockyards. Lee's disease was severe enough for him to be sent to a hospital in Portland. When Newton was released, he went to visit his son in the hospital. As he left the stockyards and breathed fresh air with the taste of freedom again, he wrote,

> I was shocked to see him [Lee] in a type of straightjacket, tied to the sides of the crib. He was standing up when I came into the room, and he began to yell because he was so happy to see me. The whole incident upset me so much that I almost did not leave. I turned my back to the cries I heard and walked out of the room, hiding my tears, and kept going. (Wesley, 1988, p. 43)

It would be almost a year and a half from that incident when Newton would see his son Lee again. Enough time would have passed that Lee would hardly recognize his father at their next meeting. Since Roy was a three-month-old baby when Newton left the family, his infant son did not have a chance to bond with him. Cecilia had the difficult task of raising two sons alone for six months in confinement without privacy or the amenities of life she used to have. This circumstance would be the first of many situations in Newton's life when he would decide to leave his family for short or long periods to create a better future for the family. After leaving the hospital, Newton went to see Mayor Earl Riley and the Portland city commissioners to thank them for helping to secure his release by writing letters of support. He informed them of his acceptance to attend Earlham College in Richmond, Indiana. He also said his goodbyes to Roy Clunes, his partner managing the Pacific College of Optometry, and to the school secretary, Mildred Birch.

Newton had never been out of the state of Oregon before, so taking the four-day train ride from Portland to Chicago with his brother was a new adventure. He sat on his suitcase much of the time because the trains were always overbooked during the war years. They traveled to Richmond, Indiana, and were taken in by a Quaker family, the Stanley Hamiltons. The dormitories at Earlham College would not open until classes began in the fall, so Newton spent the end of the summer vacation period with the Hamiltons on Quaker Hill, a large forested area just north of Richmond. The home at 10 Quaker Hill was an elegant mansion built in 1855 by Isaac Evans and used by Earlham College during the war years as a resettlement house and day camp. The Evans home was sold during the Great Depression but was purchased in 1939 by a grandson, Isaac Woodard. Isaac established the house as a center for the Friends in 1940. Newton arrived at the Evans' home during the summer of 1942. Stanley and Marie Hamilton greeted him and helped him to settle into his new lodgings. The Hamiltons lived in the house with their three children. His room might have been number one at the top of the staircase on the second floor with a view toward the expansive front lawn. In the summer of 1940, the American Friends Service Committee at Quaker Hill began to house refugees fleeing persecution by Hitler's regime. The house was not just a residence but a place where Earlham students tutored English and helped with American acculturation. Newton was a beneficiary of this noble gesture of sheltering that adhered to Quaker principles of social justice and human rights. An earlier application occurred during the Civil War when slaves would be hidden on the third floor attic room as part of the Underground Railroad network.

It was not smooth sailing for the Quakers who befriended Newton and others like him. There were hostile feelings among some of the residents of Richmond against the Quakers and the Japanese Americans. The liberal Quakers were aiding refugee Jews from Europe as well as the Japanese Americans. This letter was written September 20, 1942, to President Dennis:

Dear Sir:

I have noticed considerable unfavorable comment recently about the admission of the six American-born Japs to your college.

While it may be very true that these six students are American citizens, on the other hand they have the Jap stripe, I imagine that they are more Jap than American, and to admit them to your college now may, under the conditions, result in very unpleasant situations later on, and I wish to register my objection to their admission to your college or any other college in the United States, at this time.

Yours very truly,
Geo. N. Baker

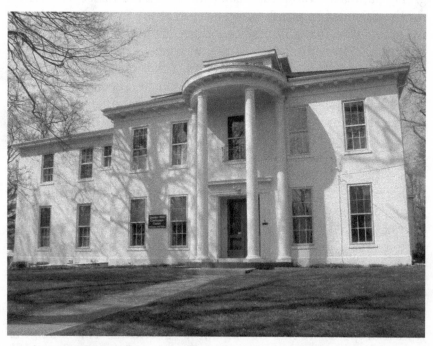

Isaac Evans' house, built in 1855, Quaker Hill, Richmond, Indiana. (Used with permission of Quaker Hill Conference Center)

A petition was circulated in Richmond to expel the Japanese American students and censure the college president for his actions. The petition quoted the local war correspondent Carroll D. Alcott, who had lived in the Far East and Japan, stating that Mr. Alcott warned that "no Japanese can be trusted except a dead one." There was even a lynch mob formed in Richmond against the Japanese Americans. The event appeared in the Richmond newspaper *The Palladium* in 1943. To the relief of the students, the mob's effort came to naught.

Despite the turbulence, Newton wrote:

The stay at Earlham College for the next two years for me were almost ideal except for the problem I was having with my eyes and being away from my family. (Wesley, 1988, p. 46)

Newton served on the Bundy Hall Council (Bundy Hall was one of the dormitories for men), played intramural football, and participated in campus life. His feelings were evident when he continued:

Here it was wartime, and it seemed unreal. I felt the privilege I had in going to college at this time during World War II. I am sure the college president, the staff, the board of directors, and the teachers did not have an easy time during this period either. (Wesley, 1988, p. 46)

Newton's Portland friend, Kermit Wilson, attempted to get permission to release Newton's family from detention at the Portland Assembly Center. Wilson was a newspaper reporter and managing editor of *This Week Magazine* in the Northwest. The magazine was a popular Sunday insert in 37 newspapers across the nation. Wilson wrote to Newton on August 5, 1942 from his home in Palo Alto, California, stating that he had spoken with Joseph Conard (a man with connections to the Western Military Command) and that:

At his suggestion, I gave him the names and approximate ages of your two children; also the name of your charming wife, Cecilia. These will be sent over to Army Headquarters for the purpose of having this information in their files when the travel permits are issued. Mr. Conard seemed to feel that there would be no trouble in taking your family with you or having them come along at a later date. He said that provision had been made to include families in the case of students. (Wilson, 1942)

Unfortunately, that was wishful thinking and planning on the part of Wilson and his colleague Mr. Conard. Newton's friends were so important to him that his son, Roy (previously mentioned), received two of his names from them: "Roy," from Roy Clunes, and "Kermit," from Kermit Wilson. Newton's older son, Lee, received Newton's first name and his middle name, "Lee," from Harry Lee Fording. His colleagues and friends were important to Newton at this time of his life. He hoped to carry them with him the rest of his life in the names of his children.

Eye Disease: Keratoconus

Before fall classes started in September 1942, Newton took advantage of his free time to go to Chicago to have his eyes examined. Newton made an appointment with Dr. Fantl, an ophthalmologist. Dr. Eric Wolfgang Fantl emigrated to the US in 1938 from Vienna with his wife, Gertrud. He practiced at 1001 W. Leland at the time of Newton's eye exam. Later Dr. Fantl taught pathology at the Northern Illinois College of Optometry and was the consultant ophthalmologist at the Chicago College of Optometry. Newton did not realize that this appointment with Dr. Fantl would set in motion events that would change the course of his life.

Dr. Fantl gave Newton a diagnosis of keratoconus, and he also gave him a prescription for a possible vision aid to help his deteriorating eyesight. He finally had a name for his affliction. Keratoconus is an eye disease where the front surface of the eye, the cornea, wrinkles, and protrudes to form a cone. It took Newton four years to discover the cause of the visual disturbances that began while he was an optometry student at North Pacific College of Optometry. Newton reported that the doctor told him, "Prepare yourself for blindness by the time you're thirty-five" in ominous tones, and he gave these instructions: "Don't lift heavy objects. Don't bend over. Your eyes might rupture!"

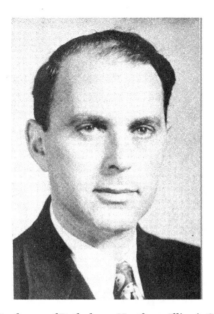

*Eric W. Fantl, MD, Professor of Pathology, Northern Illinois College of Optometry.
(NICO Yearbook, 1948)*

Dr. Fantl prescribed molded contact lenses to be fitted by an optician, Mr. Hunter. Newton's 1942 address book contained the following entry: "Mr. Hunter at Bellwood Sphere Lens Co. Phone Andover 4460." Bellwood Sphere became The House of Vision at the same Madison & Wabash location in Chicago. William Bowman observed and described the classic cone of a keratoconic eye with an ophthalmoscope in 1859. The disease "horn-shaped cornea" or keratoconus was named ten years later in 1869 by Johann Horner in his thesis. Despite its early origins, keratoconus was not well known, and many cases went uncorrected in 1940. In 1936, the Buffalo, NY, optometrist William Feinbloom was the first to utilize molded plastic scleral lenses in the treatment of keratoconus. His techniques did not move across the country to enlighten other doctors at the time. The current US incidence of keratoconus is 54 cases per 100,000 people. Statistics are not available for the 1936-1940 period, but it may be safely assumed that it was rare. Newton's complaint that he often said to people and the press was, "I visited

50 eye doctors around the country and was told that I was going blind." That indicates how difficult it was for him as a young man to be diagnosed and treated for his keratoconus.

Since school would not start until September, Newton had several weeks in August to go through the procedures of having plaster molds taken of his eyes and having shells made from the molds, which were used to create the large plastic scleral lenses to fit over the eye. These lenses created a miracle of clear vision for Newton for brief periods because the hard surface of the lenses provided a clear refracting surface that replaced the wrinkled and damaged corneal tissue of his eyes. It was miraculously encouraging, but challenging to bear the searing pain that would ensue after an hour or so of wearing the lenses. If only it could be extended and made easier must have been a thought that went through Newton's head. Several years would pass before he could act on the idea.

During his eye care visits, Newton stayed at the Quaker Friends Hostel run by Mr. Robertson Fort at 350 Belden Ave in Chicago. For $1 per day, he received a room plus three meals. Half a year later, after Newton's visits, the hostel opened officially as a Resettlement Hostel for Japanese American evacuees from the incarceration camps (February 1943).

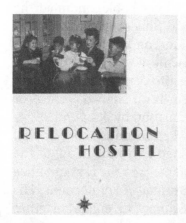

RELOCATION HOSTEL

SERVICES FOR EVACUEES

JOB PLACEMENT is part of the full-time program of the office staff of the Midwest Branch Office at 189 West Madison Street, Chicago. Evacuees are counseled, advised, and assisted in their search for employment.

Other agencies assisting evacuees are the War Relocation Authority, United States Employment Service, and Advisory Committee for Evacuees. The latter Committee is made up of representatives of over 20 religious, governmental, and private agencies interested in and offering service to evacuees in the Chicago area. Offices of the Advisory Committee are also at 189 West Madison Street.

HOUSING assistance: evacuees are aided in locating permanent residence; a staff member loaned to the Midwest Branch Office by the American Baptist Home Mission Society is engaged solely in finding suitable housing.

THROUGH INTRODUCTION to the educational, cultural, religious and social life of the neighborhood, the Hostel assists evacuees in making the necessary adjustments to the new community.

HOSPITALITY FEES

Before a job is secured: Adults—one dollar per day including three meals served at the Hostel; children (under 10 years)—fifty cents per day including three meals.

After a job has been secured: Adults—one dollar and a half per day; Children (under 10 years)—seventy-five cents per day.

1943 Quaker House for Relocation (Hostel) at 350 W. Belden, Chicago, IL, pages 1,3. (American Friends Service Committee)

When Newton returned to Earlham, he grappled with the problem that his last name had caused him over the past few years.

> ...I decided I would have my name changed - Uyesugi was just too hard to pronounce. I spent too much time trying to explain how to spell it. ... I went to an attorney and had my name changed legally, and I have never been sorry that I did. I picked the name Wesley because my mother and father were very devout Methodists. (Wesley, 1988, p. 47)

A name change to a more anglicized name would also cover his identity. Since his parents were Methodists, he thought they couldn't object to his taking the name of the founder of their faith. They did indeed object but to no avail. Newton never admitted to his family or anyone else that hiding his Japanese origin by the name change might have been a reason for his action. His stated goal for the name change was a business-related reason. He knew that patients had a hard time finding his name in the telephone book. The beginning of his thinking about changing his family name occurred when he began his optometric practice in Portland after graduating from Optometry School in 1939. A sample of his stationery letterhead was imprinted:

> DR. NEWTON K. UYESUGI (*Pronounced WES-SUGI*)
> 214 S.W. Sixth Avenue
> Portland, Oregon

He was keenly aware of the difficulty that most Caucasians would have understanding, pronouncing, or spelling his last name. He wrote:

> I knew that I would have trouble with the name, and when I started practice in Portland, I told my father about my fears. He answered, "The name has been in the family for thousands of years - it is an old Samurai name - why do you want to change it?" (Wesley, 1988, p. 47)

Newton's brother was also against the name change, saying that he was trying to hide his identity, but Newton denied that. Newton's petition for changing his surname to Wesley was granted on April 5, 1943 by the Wayne County Circuit Court Judge Gustave Hoelscher.

A few months earlier, Newton gave a speech in the Earlham College auditorium in Carpenter Hall to students and faculty on January 22, 1943. He made no mention of his immediate family or of what they went through during this period of turmoil. His "Chapel Talk" was meant to convey to his audience the loyalty and spirit of Japanese Americans as true American citizens. He wished to show some of the injustices that occurred to them after the attack at Pearl Harbor.

I am going to discuss evacuation with you today. Before I do that I want to thank you all for the manner in which Earlham — for you are Earlham — has made us feel at home here; you have done it broadmindedly and easily — you have all been swell and we wanted you to know that. There was a time when I could not discuss evacuation — it made me choke up inside of me. Time has been a great healer and now I can look at it more objectively. ...

First of all I want you to go back with me to the later 1800s in order to get a broader picture...the West was expanding and we needed labor and so we imported Chinese coolie labor and later the Japanese. The Orientals for the most part settled on the Pacific Coast. Not many Japanese came, however, until 1906-1910. At that time Japanese immigration reached its peak. In 1924 the Oriental Exclusion Act was passed so that no more Orientals would be allowed into the U.S. ...

I also want to bring out the number of Japanese in this country — many people think it runs into the millions... there are 120,000. Of that 120,000 — 80,000 are American citizens. It is a definite minority when compared to other racial stocks in the U.S. I remember figures such as 5,000,000 people of French extraction, 12-13 million negroes, and 20,000,000 of German extraction. A hundred and twenty thousand is a definite minority. When war began on DEC. 7, 1941 there was not immediate clamor for evacuation, but as time went on there were rumors of sabotage in Hawaii. Then some organizations, political groups, and businesses began to demand evacuation of the Japanese from the Coast area. ... I don't think any of us thought American citizens would be evacuated — time proved us wrong.

Events happened in rapid succession then — evacuation orders came including both aliens and citizens. We were under curfew regulations and had to stay in our residences from 8:00 PM to 6:00 AM. Travel was restricted to an area of 5 miles radius from our homes and then only for business. We had our businesses and property to dispense. I cannot help but think what a gala time the bargain hunters and the second hand dealers had. To illustrate with a few stories: a friend of mine sold his furnishings in a hotel for $750.00 — he had paid $5,000 for the furnishings during the depression; a grocer was offered $150 for a $1,500 frigidaire and $500 worth of store fixtures. A thriving business netting $1,500 a month brought $5,000. I can remember my father selling a davenport and chair, oil stove, and dining room set with 6 chairs for $55 when one article alone cost him more than that. Everybody wanted to sell and nobody would buy at a good price.

Meanwhile the Army in a few short weeks was trying to make living space for 120,000 people. Race tracks and exposition buildings were used for temporary centers.

May 5, 1942 was an eventual day which will live in my memory for that was the day I entered camp. I was among the last to leave Portland; a non-evacuee friend of ours took us in a car — on the way to the Assembly Center I can remember seeing soldiers posted on either side of the roadway. I remembered what a lovely day I thought it was; it felt good to draw the free air into my lungs, for I was soon to be behind a barbed-wire fence. When I entered camp it seemed odd to see so many people of Japanese extraction all under one roof ... 3,500 of them. I could not get used to sitting down and eating

43

on the government. ...*The people were in these temporary assembly centers for approximately 5 months.*

From the temporary assembly centers the evacuees were moved to permanent camps — Arizona, Idaho, Tule Lake and Manzanar California, Wyoming, Arkansas, and Utah were some of the locations. The people from Portland were moved to southern Idaho. Again in order to try and catch the atmosphere I am going to illustrate with a story. My aunt, who lives by herself, went with the first group of 500 for Idaho. When she reached there she found the camp was built on virgin ground and in a desolate spot; the dust storms came and obscured everything a few feet away — lights were not yet up; I guess my aunt had quite a time.

When my mother came in a few days my aunt ran to her with tears streaming down her dust-caked face — imagine a woman of 65 doing that — she just hung on to my mother and sobbed, "They've forgotten us; they have put us in a God-forsaken place!"

There are no tiled bathrooms in these centers — there are just plain necessities. Everything has been built from the ground up — sanitation systems, lights (there were no lights at first) — water (no hot water at first), etc. The caucasian personnel of these camps have been working night and day to arrange for these things, but it takes time....

Evacuation was unique in that there has been no precedent for it in the history of the United States — it is the first time in our history that we have moved American citizens of a particular racial background without due process of law.

Some believe it is a dangerous precedent since the next time it could be that people of any particular racial background might be moved. Therefore test cases have sprung up in our courts — too late to stop evacuation but to prove the rights of citizens and the principles upon which our nation stands and for which we are fighting today.

I want to get across to you the idea that the Americans of Japanese ancestry are trying with their hearts and souls to prove they are American citizens. ...

When I first came here someone said, "School is the closest thing I know to Utopia." I like the way you have stood up during these turbulent times; ...carry that Utopia with you into the world. Don't stop practicing it. I want you to realize the value of citizenship; don't take it for granted. I have watched the American citizens of Japanese ancestry going through so much to prove that they are Americans in spirit and in thought, and not because of birth, to let you do so.

In closing I want to point out the brightest symbol of all in this auditorium — the flag. I often like to think of what it represents. The red for valor and the blood of those who have fought and died for the principles of our nation; the white for hope, purity, and charity; the white stars on a blue background for the stars in heaven. (Wesley, 1943)

Newton had to finance his life away from his family. There were college tuition and rooming costs, travel, and daily living expenses. He had saved money from his work as an optometrist in Portland, but the main source of income were monthly payments from the Villa House hotel, which his parents owned. Mrs. Cora Oliver, a family friend and a friend to many Japanese students, took over the management of the hotel during the war years and returned it to them after the war. That act of kindness was rare and the Uyesugi/Wesley family has been eternally grateful. Cora sent the monthly rental payments to Newton so that he could live through those years. Cora married Clarence E. Oliver in 1928 when she was 18. She did missionary work in Japan, and upon returning, joined the Japanese American Methodist Episcopal church in Portland with her husband. They developed close relationships with the church community. Clarence was a school teacher, and in 1941, was the Teacher's Union President. When war broke out in 1942, he wrote Governor Sprague as a non-Japanese voice to convince him that they were "useful and loyal citizens." Oliver recommended that Sprague appoint committees of prominent citizens "to serve in a guardianship capacity for the people of Japanese blood residing in our state." As a couple, the Olivers worked to assist young Japanese Americans to continue their education and obtain financing to attend colleges through the Quaker network.

While Newton created a new life as a student, there was the harsh daily reality of imprisonment for his wife, Cecilia, and his two sons in the barbed wired and rifle guarded camp at Minidoka, Idaho. Cecilia took it upon herself to write a plea for early release to Mr. Elmer Shirrell, the War Relocation Supervisor in the first regional field office of the WRA (War Relocation Authority). The Chicago WRA office was opened January 1943. Cecilia wrote May 1943 to Mr. Shirrell as a Wesley, stating that "my husband has legally changed his name of Uyesugi to Wesley. The reason being that, Uyesugi, being such a hard name to pronounce and for our Caucasian American friends to remember. Also, for business reasons, he has changed his name." She described her plight as having two young children and being alone at Minidoka since her husband was studying "pre-medics" at Earlham College. In order to qualify for release, she needed to prove that she could support herself and she stated:

> *I have worked in his office for three years as, Receptionist-Technician. I would prefer something in that line but I doubt if you have such an opening available.*
>
> *I am confident and anxious to try and learn any other field provided that I am able to support myself and my two children.*
>
> *As to my other abilities, I am able to sew, I have worked in a glove factory, using a power sewing machine. I have worked in a grocery store as clerk. ...*
>
> *I am more than anxious to send my husband through school and to unite as a family again.* (Wesley, C., 1943)

Mr. Shirrell wrote back on June 8, 1943, stating that no jobs were available in Chicago as receptionist-technician in an optometric office, but that her "experience as a power sewing machine operator ... would have no difficulty in getting a job in this city." He goes on to describe the details of the work involved and pay. He also mentions daycare for children in Chicago so that she could be accommodated to go to work. He recommends that her husband come to Chicago to "locate housing for you and the children" (Shirrell, 1943,).

During the Christmas break in December 1943 at Earlham College, Newton arranged to visit his family nearly 18 months after his release from the Portland Assembly Center in July 1942. He realized that at the end of the Second World War, the camps would be closed by the War Relocation Authority. Cecilia's letter to the WRA helped in obtaining an early release. Newton started to make plans and prepare his family for relocation. He had fallen in love with the city of Chicago during his travels from Portland to Richmond and decided that it was the ideal place for him to settle his family. Newton took the train from Chicago to Pocatello, Idaho, where he waited for the next train to reach Jerome, Idaho, the next morning. He would then take a bus to the Minidoka concentration camp at Hunt, Idaho. He tried to rent a hotel room in Pocatello to spend the night, but there were no vacancies. He had to sleep in the train station. The train that traveled the 110 miles between Pocatello to Jerome was called "The Goose," and Newton remarked, "the train was well named because it would rattle and waddle like a goose. Any moment you expected it to take off." When he arrived, he said, "The camp was in the wilderness - desolate, dusty and, in this case, real muddy after the rains." Newton had no idea of the reality of the dismal daily conditions that his family had endured during his absence and freedom at Earlham College. Newton had to confront the sad fate of his family after a nearly two-year absence. How different this reality was from the Earlham College environment that he left.

Newton missed eighteen critical developmental bonding months with his two boys, Lee and Roy. Lee was a 17-month-old toddler, and Roy was two months old when Newton left. He also left his distraught 25-year-old wife imprisoned in the animal stockyards in Portland. Lee was last seen clinging to his hospital crib, crying for him not to go. Lee had grown into an almost unrecognizable 3-year-old whose second and third birthdays he had missed. His second son, Roy, was an infant when Newton left. Roy had grown into a timid and frightened 1½-year old toddler when he visited at Christmas. Cecilia had to bear the loneliness of separation from her husband. She did have some support of her mother and in-laws nearby in the squalid, crowded quarters that was their home in the bleak desert. For Cecilia, the two-year separation from Newton was the longest in their married life.

The first family person Newton met on his arrival at Minidoka was his aunt Suye Uyesugi Shiozaki, Newton's father's sister, who

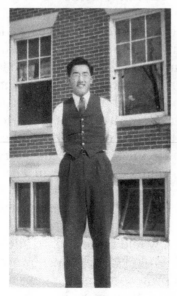
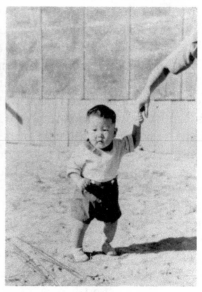
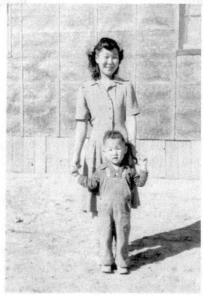

TOP LEFT: Newton Wesley at Earlham College, 1944. TOP RIGHT: Roy Wesley at Minidoka, 1943. BOTTOM: Cecilia and Lee Wesley at Minidoka barrack, 1943. (Roy Wesley personal collection)

cried tears of joy to see him. She said, "America has forgotten us, and we are buried in the wilderness" as they laboriously walked knee-deep in the mud to the family barrack. Newton met his family for the first time after two and a half years. He wrote about the meeting, saying, "It was unreal. Lee, my older son, was clinging to Grandma, and he was shy and appeared not to know me, which I am sure he didn't. Roy had a shock of hair – jet black – and they both looked immense to me because of the time that had passed. Everyone had tears in their eyes. We had a great deal to discuss." The tears that flowed were mixed tears of the joy of reunion with the sadness of isolation.

There was much to be discussed as Newton told the family the news that they would be released from Minidoka in January 1944. Preparations had to be made for reintegration into normal American life. In Newton's mind, a return to the Pacific Northwest was not an option because of the prejudice encountered there before they left.

It took years for a healing reintegration of Japanese American families into mainstream American life. It was a complicated process for many former internees trying to re-establish what they remembered as their pre-war lives. The U.S. government slowly recognized the errors made in taking away the freedom of Japanese Americans. President Gerald Ford, in 1976, signed Proclamation 4417, recognizing the end of the internment camps and stating, "We now know what we should have known then, not only that evacuation was wrong, but Japanese Americans were and are loyal Americans." A reparations bill was passed in Congress that same year, the bicentennial of the United States. Richard Reeves in his book *Infamy: The Shocking Story of the Japanese American Internment in World War II* states that in the 1982 Commission report "Personal Justice Denied," that "Perhaps the most significant sentences of the report were: 'In sum, Executive Order 9066 was not justified by military necessity, and the decisions that followed from it—exclusion, detention, the ending of detention, and the ending of exclusion—were not founded on military considerations. The broad historical causes that shaped these decisions were race prejudice, war hysteria, and a failure of political leadership.'"

As citizens, we need to be mindful of racial prejudice, profiling, and discrimination that led to the internment of honest American citizens. Without vigilance, it can happen again.

6 STARTING OVER

Newton did not return to Earlham for the fall semester of 1943 but chose to look for employment in Chicago and to look for places to settle his family. He rented apartment #103 at 430 West Diversey on the north side of Chicago just two blocks from Lincoln Park and Lake Michigan. The apartment building was next door to the famous Brewster Building, built in 1893 as the Lincoln Park Palace. The Brewster was home to former Illinois Governor John Altgeld after his tenure, and Charlie Chaplin was said to live in the penthouse while filming in Chicago. Newton reveled in the vibrant life of Chicago, taking buses and the "L" one of the Chicago Surface Lines (the CSL preceded the CTA, Chicago Transit Authority). A trip on the CSL cost ten cents in 1943, and transfers were available. The extensive network of trains, streetcars, and buses of Chicago allowed Newton access to all areas of the city. He gave notice to Earlham College that he would be leaving and requested that his credits be transferred to Loyola University in Chicago.

Newton decided that he liked Chicago as a city and a place for opportunities in the future. It had excitement, energy, and dynamism that was lacking in Portland. The faster pace of diverse people walking to work and riding the "L" around the Loop invigorated him. He enjoyed his quiet time and the beauty of the college campus at Earlham but felt that Richmond, Indiana, was too small a town in which to do business. His brother, Edward, remained on campus to finish his studies and graduated from Earlham while Newton said goodbye to his friends and teachers who had supported him during the past couple of years. Ed preferred the quiet life of Earlham and Indiana small towns, as proven by his marriage to a Quaker classmate, Ruth Ann Farlow, and moving to her family's small town, Paoli, Indiana, for the remainder of his life.

Newton faced another abrupt change. He had become comfortable being a student involved with campus activities. Now he needed to become a father, husband, and provider again. He had to find living quarters for the family and get a job to support the family. There was not much time to get those things done since his family was scheduled to leave Minidoka January 29, 1944.

Newton searched for a home to buy, but properties were scarce during the war years. He found one in Rogers Park, but the house was sold to someone who placed a higher bid. He settled for a rental apartment in a mostly Jewish area that was not hostile to Japanese Americans. Josephine Edelstein sold her furniture and her lease on the two-bedroom greystone flat at 1340 W. Douglas Blvd to Newton and asked him "Do you know you are moving into a Jewish neighborhood?"

"Yes, I don't mind. I noticed the kosher delicatessen and other stores. I like the neighborhood," he replied.

Newton told his sons that he preferred Jewish neighborhoods because he knew that the education standards would be high.

Providing a good education for their children was always an important expectation Newton and Cecilia had. That their children would go to college was taken for granted. Even though they were born second-generation Americans, they retained the non-verbal disciplined communication common to many Japanese families, inherited through generations.

When Newton left Earlham College to settle the family, he transferred his credits to Loyola University but never finished his degree. He had enrolled thinking that he would eventually get a medical doctor's degree, but that was put on hold. He said that his mother wanted him to be a medical doctor; however "he couldn't stand the sight of blood." The seed that his mother planted in his mind remained dormant but was a persistent reminder of a dutiful son's obligation to his mother. He fulfilled his filial duty at the age of 59 when he received a MD research degree from Osaka University based on work that he and his team did at Wesley-Jessen.

Newton's wife and children left Minidoka by train on January 29, 1944, and arrived in Chicago, where he greeted them at Union Station to take them to their new home. Compared with the sparse, cramped barrack room in Minidoka, the spacious first floor two-bedroom apartment was luxurious for the family. Instead of dry, dusty desert land that turned to mud and ice in the winter, there was a large park with trees just a block away. There was the luxury of a warm bathroom with plumbing inside the apartment instead of walking to the common toilets and wash areas. There was the freedom to just walk out the front door and go wherever you wanted without being watched by armed guards with rifles and surrounded by barbed wire fences.

Chicago in wartime 1944 was still a vibrant city reflecting the past decade's sins of Al Capone and other mobsters and the struggle to emerge out of the Great Depression. Soldiers on furlough came to Chicago seeking relief on their break from training or battlefronts in Europe and Asia at the many venues provided for their entertainment. Free transportation was provided on the buses, subways, and the "L" and Chicago's GI service centers offered free lodging and other services. Some 6,000 girls came into the Chicago dance halls like the Aragon Ballroom. Some worked at the free burlesque stages for the GIs. Chicago honored the fallen soldiers with plaques posted with their names and gold stars on many blocks of the city to remember the neighborhood boys who sacrificed their lives in the war. Blue stars in windows signified that a family member was in the military. Older men who were not in the war and women joined the newly spawned war effort industries like the ones to build more planes for the Air Force. Chicagoans pitched in to help the war effort through their work in factories producing parachutes, torpedoes, and canned rations. Food was scarce and rationed to families. Bakeries sold out of bread quickly, and meat was distributed every other day. Gasoline for cars was rationed. People collected bottles and scrap metal to help the war effort.

Chicago was and is a city of distinct ethnic neighborhoods. Newton chose to settle in a stable Jewish area on the west side of Chicago. There were small clusters of Japanese American communities located on the south side of Chicago at Hyde Park, Kenwood, and along Clark Street on the north side. He instinctively followed his father's pattern of not clinging to comfortable ethnic neighborhoods but branching out to integrate into mainstream America.

Monroe College of Optometry (Illinois College of Optometry)

Newton realized that he had to make a living to support his family. His experience teaching and operating the Pacific College of Optometry in Portland was an excellent credential to help get him a teaching position. He spoke to Dr. Eugene Freeman, the dean of the Chicago

College of Optometry (later merged into the Illinois College of Optometry). The dean said that the college didn't have many students because of the war, and he was not hiring new faculty. He suggested that Newton should apply for a teaching job at Monroe College of Optometry. Monroe College President Reuben Seid, MD, interviewed Newton with the result that Newton received and accepted a job offer. The Monroe College of Optometry was founded in 1936 as the Midwestern College of Optometry by Dr. Seid. The name was changed and merged into the Illinois College of Optometry in 1955.

The 1942 Chicago Classified Directory lists the Monroe College of Optometry at 180 N. Wacker Drive, Chicago, with a telephone number of CENtrl-3444. The College of Optometry occupied offices in a six-story building along Wacker Drive near the Chicago River. The building was built in 1923 and stands today with the same first-floor window design as seen in the 1944 photo of Dr. Wesley with Monroe College faculty.

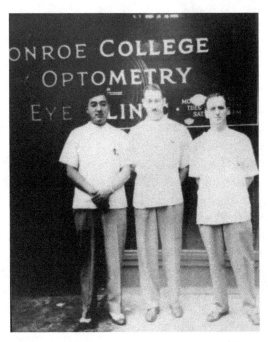

Monroe College of Optometry, 1944: Dr. Newton K. Wesley, Dr Maurice Charlens, Dr. Dan Davis. Photo taken in front of first level of 180 N. Wacker building. (Roy Wesley personal collection)

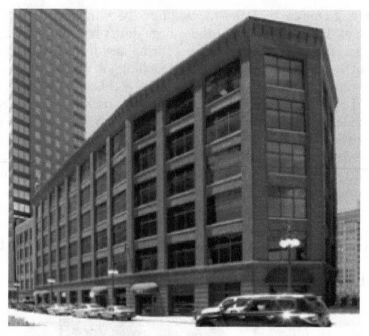

1944 home of the Monroe College of Optometry: 180 N. Wacker Drive, Chicago. The building in 1971. (Roy Wesley personal collection)

In addition to the Monroe College schedule of teaching classes in clinical optometry, anatomy, physiology, pathology, visual fields, and orthoptics, Newton also worked at Northwestern University's Wesley Memorial Hospital Clinic. He wrote, "I saw more pathology than I had in all the years that I had practiced." Intense work schedules were not new to him. There was a cost to his visual health when he reported, "I would drive up and down the Outer Drive and at night I noticed that the lights were getting dimmer and dimmer and there was greater polyopia [multiple images]." He further wrote, "I began to feel very sorry for myself again, but I was not going to let it get to me. I must solve the problem. I realized I had to face the problem." He did face his problem with the help of two students enrolled in his classes.

Newton's parents were released from Minidoka and arrived in Chicago in July 1944. He was looking to house the family, and he searched for hotels in Chicago to buy for his parents to run. Newton's father disagreed with Newton about where to resettle after the war. He preferred to go back to Portland, where he still had a property waiting for him. Mrs. Cora Oliver played a significant role in saving the family from financial ruin. She took over one of Harry Uyesugi's hotels in Portland to protect it from greedy bargain hunters taking advantage. She managed the Villa House hotel for him until he returned. Mrs. Cora Oliver was one of many courageous Americans who saw through the propaganda of the day. She and her husband, Clarence Oliver, considered the treatment of Japanese Americans to be unjust and was willing to do something to help. When Harry Uyesugi declared that he wanted to return to Portland, the War Relocation Authority began to allow Japanese Americans back to the West Coast. Newton provided the necessary funds for his parents to return to Portland to continue their life managing hotels there. He gave his father five thousand dollars, which was all the cash he had left.

The relocation period was one of flux and confusion for many members of Japanese American families. Each individual tried to integrate into a new life after two to three years of forced imprisonment. There was no easy path to integration in a society that had formed strong anti-Japanese prejudices. Those feelings were not easily turned off once the war was over, and words did not have to be spoken to interpret the glaring glances and stern stares. Japanese Americans looked like the former enemy. Newton's brother Edward and his mixed-marriage family had a difficult time settling down and lived with Newton and his family for a while. Cecilia's brother, Ed Sasaki, also came to live with the family for some time after he served his time in the US Army 442nd Regiment. He saw action in the South of France and Northern Italy and helped to save the Lost Battalion in the Argonne. Ed learned a new trade in electronics, servicing radios and TVs at a school in Chicago. The home at 1430 W. Douglas Boulevard became a place of refuge for family members trying to reestablish themselves after the war.

Newton thought he might have a solution for his worsening eye problem. He had the experience of improved vision using the large molded corneal scleral lenses during his previous summer visit to Chicago. He wrote:

In the back of my mind, I was thinking about finding someone who would know how to make contact lenses and do research to solve my problem. If I had a hernia, what is more logical than to use a truss, even though it would be on the eye. In this instance, it was a truss to shape the front of my eye – the cornea. When I discussed this with doctors, they would pooh-pooh the idea that it wouldn't work and said that I would go blind faster, that I would injure the cornea, and the process could cause scar tissue to develop. I certainly could not find a contact lens maker or anyone who would show me how to make them. (Wesley, 1988, p. 54)

Despite the discouraging advice he received, Newton talked about his ideas for improving contact lenses with his classes at Monroe College of Optometry. From those discussions, he inspired two students to help him in researching the creation of better lenses. His collaborators were George N. Jessen of Chicago and Valentine J. Kuehn from Milwaukee, Wisconsin. George was exempted from military service because he was afflicted by polio as a child and was left with a lifelong limp. George worked as an optician at Miller Optical Company, where he was the foreman. Val was also an optician working at Riggs Optical. Both men were enrolled full time at Monroe, kept their jobs, and graduated in June 1945. All three men had families to support by working at their jobs in addition to attending Monroe College of Optometry and being engaged in a contact lens research project. George Nissen Jessen, born of a Danish American father and German American mother in 1916, was married to Lillian Dempsey Jessen, a fiery, red-headed Irish descendant, and the couple had one son, Michael. George became interested in optics because his father was blind (Bowden and Gasson, 2006, p. 14). George senior must have had visual problems later in life since his occupation in the 1920 US Census was a coffee broker and then he became an insurance agent according to the 1930 Census. Val Kuehn was 17 years older than Newton and married to Myrtle Kuehn. They had a 14-year-old daughter, Lorainne. Val worked as a superintendent at Riggs Optical while attending school. They did their contact lens research in the evenings, weekends, and on holidays in the basement of Bertha Jessen's apartment building at 5218 North Kenmore in Chicago's Edgewater district. Bertha was George's widowed mother. The additional contact lens project became too much for Val Kuehn to manage when he began his optometric practice. He dropped out of the project and left George and Newton to carry on with their endeavor.

In a conversation with George's son, Michael Jessen, he reported, "They would heat up sheets of plastic to make scleral lenses to help Newton's keratoconus. The plastic sheets were methyl methacrylate rectangles that they would heat up on the third floor where we lived and run them downstairs to the basement where the press was. They heated the plastic sheets outside, even in the winter, to avoid the fumes." George made molds of Newton's eyes for the scleral lenses. They made Michael a guinea pig at an early age and made molds of his eyes to fit contacts. Michael sent Roy Wesley two scleral lenses from that time when they produced lenses in those early days.

Newton and George learned fundamental procedures of making contact lenses from plastic rather than glass. They learned about

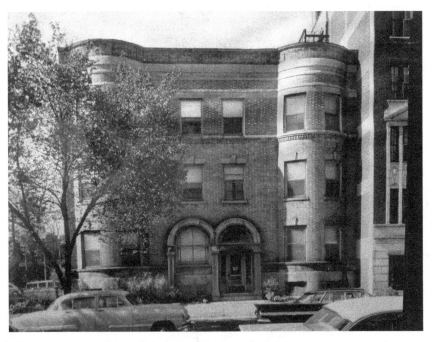

5218 N Kenmore, Chicago, Illinois, 1957. Site of Newton Wesley and George Jessen's experiments to produce contact lenses. (Roy Wesley personal collection)

lens optics and formulas for determining the power of the lenses, grinding and mold making, polishing the surface, and other details in the manufacture of the lenses. In a 1970 published newsletter from Wesley-Jessen, Newton expanded on this early time period. He said that:

> Val Kuehn, Dr. Jessen and I used an old fashioned foot pedal type sewing machine to hack out contact lenses. Though the machine had been converted into a spindle it remained equipment of the simplest kind. It did, however enable us to solve most of the problems of making a contact lens–all except the final polishing step which was resolved by James Kawabata, an engineer.

Finding a solution to the polishing step required searching outside their connections. Newton spoke to a colleague, and he recommended that he talk to James Kawabata, who later helped design instrumentation for the company and solved the immediate problem of polishing the lenses. It was a simple chemical modification using stannous oxide (SnO) for the polishing solution instead of the stannic oxide (SnO_2). It was the latter chemical that provided the proper polishing finish. Mr. Kawabata later developed a micrometer reading attachment (US Patent 2,6181,94A, 1952) and a torque meter (US Patent 3,163,037, 1964). Solving simple or complex problems created excitement for these two men. Their collaboration in the apartment building basement led to their working together in an optometric practice and the beginnings of a contact lens manufacturing company. Newton and George worked for three years in the basement of Bertha Jessen's Kenmore Avenue apartment building.

The third job that Newton took on while teaching at Monroe College was to open his optometric practice. There were only three office spaces available at the time he was looking. He chose a space in the Mallers Building at 59 East Madison in downtown Chicago, just a block away from Michigan Avenue. His wife, Cecilia, also attended Monroe College of Optometry and joined him part-time in practice. Later, George Jessen entered the practice with them.

George Jessen said that to combat the prejudice of the time in 1945, he would often tell people that his partner was "Korean" to hide Newton's real background and to offset any prejudice that people held at that time. George's son Michael Jessen related that story to Roy Wesley. Another way of covering his identity was the name change that Newton undertook while at Earlham College. He changed his given family name, Uyesugi, to a more anglicized name of "Wesley." Newton never admitted that hiding his Japanese origin by the name change might have been a reason for his action. His stated goal for the name change was a business-related reason.

A year after World War II ended, there were racial innuendos, as demonstrated by an August 30, 1946, Acme Roto Service press release photo with the news story lead pasted on the back. Biased comments were on the back of a press photo of Cecilia and Newton at their optometric clinic doing visual training.

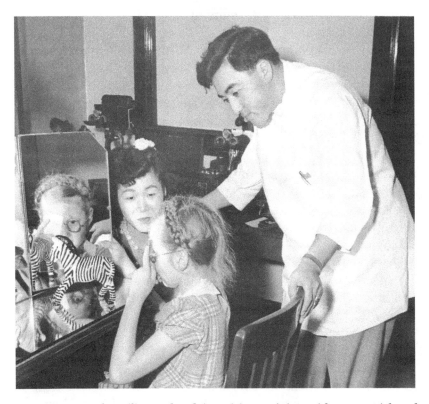

1946, Newton and Cecilia Wesley doing vision training with young girl at the American Vision Training Center, Chicago, Illinois. (Photograph from the collection of Dr. Jenna Williams Wesley)

Acme Roto Service news story line: Newton K. Uyesugi is a graduate of North Pacific Optometry College at Portland, Ore. He later attended Earlham, a Quaker College in Indiana, and Loyola, a Catholic college in Chicago. He teaches at Monroe College of Optometry in Chicago, where he met his wife, then one of his students. They were separated for two years when she was sent to a relocation camp in Idaho. On her release, Mrs. Uyesugi re-entered Monroe College and earned her diploma. Now she is associated with her husband in his work. Here, Mrs. Uyesugi gives corrective optical exercises to a little girl, while her husband watches. (Acme Roto Service Press Release August 30, 1946, sent to Chicago newspapers for distribution)

An obvious error of the text refers to Newton as "Uyesugi." He established himself as Dr. Newton K. Wesley, and he had already legally changed his name in 1943. The Monroe College of Optometry Faculty gave him a "Dr. Newton K. Wesley" listing at the school. Another error was that he did not meet his wife at Monroe College but in Seattle. The most revealing item is on the back of the photograph. There is a handwritten line in pencil stating: "Japs in US Chgo Jap Colony."

Newton had some of his equipment from his practice in Portland and was able to buy used equipment from other optometrists. For the first six months of the optometric practice, George Jessen continued to work as an optician at Miller Optical Company. They saved money from their jobs to invest in their project developing contact lenses.

The family was united, and Newton was busy outside the home with his three jobs. Cecilia managed the house while helping at the clinic. When the opportunity came for her mother, Yae Sasaki, to live with the family, she successfully integrated into the home. Mother-in-law Sasaki was released from Minidoka on September 20, 1944. Before coming to Chicago, she tried working in New York City as a house-maid for a family living in a 5th Avenue apartment at 77th Street. It must have been a shock for her to come from the quiet, desolate desert of eastern Idaho to bustling sophisticated New York with her limited English skills. She remained in the Wesley household for the rest of her life, helping to raise his family.

After Cecilia's death in 1973, Mrs. Sasaki continued to live with and help raise Newton's second family. She was the rock of family stability, preparing multiple breakfasts to accommodate everyone's waking and departure schedule. She often made many meals to accommodate working schedules and looked after the children.

7 BUSINESS BUILDING IN CHICAGO

Newton and George were pioneers in the development of contact lenses during the 1940s, when the concept of wearing them was mostly unknown. The available lenses were large, uncomfortable glass or plastic lenses that covered almost the entire surface of the eye. As with many inventions, the time was ripe for innovation.

Some of Newton's optometry school students became lifelong colleagues and friends. George Jessen graduated from Monroe College of Optometry in 1945, along with Val Kuehn, Samuel Lane (later friend, company supporter, and insurer of contact lenses), Orlando Giraldi, and Chester Nowak (supporters of WJ and NERF). Albert Odey was a student of Newton's and graduated a year earlier in 1944. Al became a board member on Newton's enterprises, including the American Optometric Center and the National Eye Research Foundation. He became the founder and CEO of Morrison Institute of Technology and a lifelong friend.

Newton realized that trying to compete against the more than 2,000 local licensed Chicago optometrists to make a living and accomplish his contact lens research goals was not realistic. He decided that his practice would be a specialty clinic to handle difficult, complicated, and time-consuming cases that doctors did not want to treat or would prefer to refer to specialists. Newton resigned his teaching position at Monroe College to spend full time in the new clinic established with George Jessen.

The clinic opened in 1945 and was named the American Vision Center. Newton's patriotic fervor continued in his need to be "all American" in the naming of his businesses. The deadliest global conflict, World War II, had just ended in Europe in the spring of 1945 while the war against Japan ended in the fall. The many years of fear, prejudice, and discrimination against Japanese Americans did not disappear as quickly as the war ended. Newton lived in an environment of potential suspicion by new patients and people in business. Partnering with George Jessen provided a protective cover for him during the transition period to peace and into the company's future development. Newton's engaging personality and charisma did much to win people over as well.

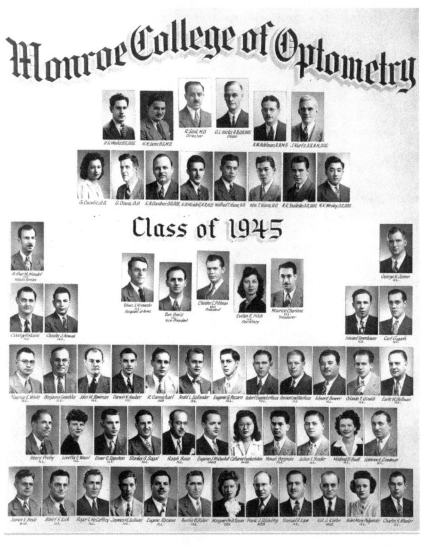

Dr. Newton K. Wesley is shown with the faculty on the second row, far right. Recruits and associates from the 1945 class to his company over time were George Jessen (3rd row, right), Orlando Giraldi (5th row, right), Sam Lane (bottom row, right) and Val Kuehn (bottom row, right). (Used with permission of the Illinois College of Optometry)

The clinic tended to specialize in vision training. Vision training corrects eye motor and nerve dysfunctions resulting in strabismus (cross-eyes, wide eyes), amblyopia (lazy eye), eye and motor dysfunctions, and visual perception problems. The clinic treated mostly children, but also some adults.

Within three years, the clinic practice expanded in numbers of patients and staff, as seen in the photograph below. In truth, not all shown worked in the clinic. Joseph Cinefro and Chuck Nishimura were workers at Plastic Contact Lens but were recruited for the picture.

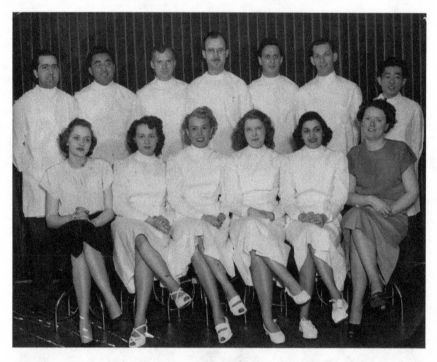

American Vision Center, Ca 1948. Back row: Joseph Cinefro, Newton K. Wesley, George Jessen, Arthur Mandel, John Groppi, Ed Wilkowski, Chuck Nishimura. Front row: Marilyn Jensen, Delores Bromar, Bette Bagnell, Ann Moss, Beverly Argenzio, Lillian Jessen. 59 E. Madison St., Suite 415. (Roy Wesley personal collection)

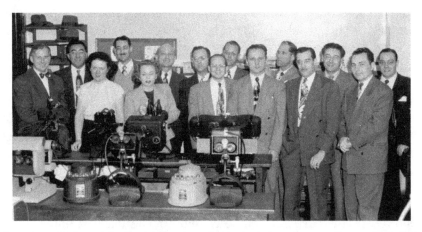

American Optometric Center postgraduate training course, Ca 1946. Left to right: George Jessen, Newton Wesley, Lillian Jessen, unidentified doctor, Bette Bagnel, other doctors in the course. 59 E Madison St., Suite 415.
(Roy Wesley personal collection)

America was looking toward the future with optimism and hoping for economic recovery. Many returning soldiers used the GI Bill (the Serviceman's Readjustment Act of 1944) to pay for tuition and expenses to attend colleges or trade schools. A year after the opening of the American Vision Center in 1945, Newton established The American Optometric Center (incorporated September 16, 1946), offering post-graduate courses for doctors of optometry under the GI Bill of the Veteran's Administration. Optometry schools across the country and in Chicago were flooded with veterans entering the field. These newly minted doctors were eager to expand the knowledge base and get practical experience in their new-found field. Doctors often graduated after one year of optometry school, and they often needed to practice skills not fully developed in school. According to the Center's promotional material, they offered post-graduate courses for optometrists in "advanced visual analysis & procedures, visual training & visual fields, and contact lens fitting." For doctors' assistants and technicians, they provided courses in "visual training, visual analysis checking, chaining and typing, physiology of finds, mechanics of the 21-point exam, contact lens grinding, dispensing and retinoscopy." "Chaining" is learning to analyze tasks in small steps to gain a skill. Newton and the staff taught these courses after a workday of seeing patients in the clinic. The photo of the group of doctors below exemplifies their enthusiasm and vigor (just one of many pictures of the hundreds of doctors who went through the postgraduate classes).

The need for the American Optometric Training Center diminished over a few years as the GIs integrated into society and the benefit program ended. The Center transitioned into training doctors in the fitting of contact lenses to support the contact lens manufacturing business. The American Vision Training Center transitioned into Wesley-Jessen with George taking over the clinical practice and seeing patients. Newton managed the contact lens manufacturing business, which was initially incorporated Plastic Contact Lens Company (1947), followed by the corporate name change to The Plastic Contact Lens Company (1948), and finally, Wesley-Jessen, Inc. (1959). Establishing a

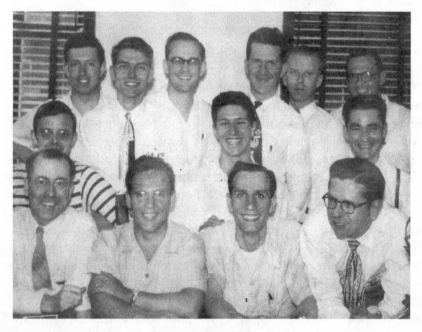

Post graduate optometrists who had taken the American Optical Center's courses, Ca 1948, Chicago. L to R, front row: Art Copes, John Kurzara, Frank Gianfriddo, Calvin M. King. 2nd Row: Russell Dorland, Roy Freeman, Frank Cribbs. 3rd Row: Paul Freeman, Wallis Reagin, Phillip Myhre, Charles R. Moyers, Art Moen, Edward Jones. (Roy Wesley personal collection)

contact lens manufacturing company was the beginning of a revolution in eye care in the United States. The clinical practice was re-organized as Jessen Wesley & Associates and grew to a staff of many doctors and technicians located in several Chicago offices. Wesley-Jessen grew to a medium-sized manufacturing company of over 600 employees up to the company's sale to Schering-Plough in 1981.

Another man working on making smaller lenses from the large scleral lenses about the same time was Kevin Tuohy, who was born in 1921 in Hasbrouck, New Jersey, four years after Newton Wesley. Coincidentally, he was afflicted by polio as a child, as was Newton's partner, George Jessen. Despite his handicap, Kevin was hired by Theodore Obrig in 1939 to assist in making the large glass and plastic scleral lenses in New York. In 1947, a portion of the large plastic scleral lens broke off, and Kevin Tuohy modified the lens into a smaller round lens. He smoothed the edges of the lens and tried fitting it on a patient. He tried the smaller designed lenses on several patients and then applied for a patent in 1948. A patent on Tuohy's lens design made of polymethyl methacrylate (PMMA) plastic was granted in 1950. His patent was later modified by George Butterfield in Portland, Oregon, to produce better alignment of the lens to the cornea. In a twist of serendipitous fate, it was Kevin Touhy's brother-in-law who fitted Newton with new scleral contact lenses in Chicago. Newton noted that "I could not wear them without abrasions. I knew they held promise, and the corneal lenses would certainly be an aid to alleviate the weight on the cornea when I went to conform the eye to the lens."

Curiously, a discovery was made searching through Newton's 1936 scrapbook assembled when he was 18 years old and about to begin optometry school. He had cut out an article from the Portland newspaper describing Dr. William Feinbloom's "new form-fitting eyeglass," or contact lens "worn under the eyelids." He must have forgotten about this clipping through the years as he never referred to it, but perhaps its influence was buried in his mind. 1936 is the year Feinbloom introduced plastic lenses, making them lighter and more convenient. The initial lenses were a combination of glass and plastic. In 1940, German optometrist Heinrich Wöhlk produced plastic lenses, based on experiments performed during the 1930s.

The Butterfield patent was filed in 1950 and granted in 1951. Both of these patents were part of a long-lasting patent fight, which Wesley-Jessen settled out of court, with the result that WJ obtained royalty rights from the patents. Kevin Tuohy moved to the Los Angeles area and opened a contact lens practice that had many Hollywood stars as clients. A tragic outcome was Kevin Tuohy's death by suicide in 1968 at the age of 47.

Newton Wesley wrote in his 1953 *Contact Lens Practice*, "...

> Dr. A. Eugen Fick of Zurich, Switzerland, made known results of experiments in which he used contact lenses as a refractive device. He experimented with rabbits and cadavers by taking casts of their eyes with plaster of Paris, then having glass lenses blown over these molds. After deriving satisfactory results with these experiments, he asked Prof. Abbe, an associate of Carl Zeiss, to make lenses for him. Although the results were unsuccessful, he continued with his experiments, endeavoring to solve clinical problems that baffle men in the field even today. He contributed much to the advancement of contact lenses. (Wesley & Jessen, 1953, p. 7)

It is interesting to note that he was the first to use the terminology "contact lens" (Kontact Brille). Ernst Karl Abbe (1840 –1905) was a German physicist, optical scientist, entrepreneur, and social reformer. Together with Otto Schott and Carl Zeiss, he laid the foundation of modern optics. Abbe developed numerous optical instruments. Professor Abbe was also a co-owner of Carl Zeiss AG. In history, Abbe's optical work and discoveries, such as the mathematical formulas for the achromatic lens, overshadowed the work that he did in contact lenses.

Adolf Eugen Fick published his work "Contactbrille" in the journal *Archiv für Augenheilkunde* in March 1888. Adolf Fick made glass scleral contact shells that sat on the white of the eye (the sclera), and he filled the space between the cornea and the glass shell with a dextrose solution. These blown glass scleral lenses were the only form of early "contact lenses" until the 1930's when PMMA (also known as Perspex/Plexiglas) was developed. Using PMMA allowed for plastic scleral lenses to be manufactured for the first time.

In 1946, Newton and George moved the equipment from the basement of the apartment building to the same building where Newton first established his clinical practice, 59 East Madison Ave, in Chicago's Loop. Newton's networking with Paul Smythe led to a company in which Mr. Smythe had an investment, Kolograph of Indianapolis, founded by Mr. Kohlmeyer. Kolograph manufactured 16-mm projectors, but the engineering connection helped Newton develop many items used in the manufacturing process for contact lenses such as a diameter gauge and an instrument to measure the lenses' curvature Wesley-Jessen manufactured and named the Contactometer. WJ's first employee Chuck Nishimura developed a bevel on the edge of the lens, which added significantly to wearability and comfort and became known in the industry as the "CN" bevel. For many years, students taking the National Boards for Optometry qualification faced the question, "What is the CN bevel?" The correct multiple choice answer was a variant of a plus lenticular design or an anterior blend to thin the edge of a minus lens. To this day, almost no one knows that "CN" refers to Chuck Nishimura, the design's originator.

Newton wrote:

> There were many systems that we instituted that were original and patentable, such as the Bonnet system, a way of making contact lenses and holding the lens blank precisely, eliminating prisms, developing glasslike optics, methods of making the lenses to size with lens punches, methods of making toric contact lenses to correct astigmatism, bifocal contact lenses, contact lenses with graduated curves, and so on. As far as I know, we were the first to bring computers into the ophthalmic field. (Wesley, 1988, p. 64)

Newton incorporated The Plastic Contact Lens Company (PCL) on June 25, 1948, as an Illinois corporation. The first contact lenses that the Plastic Contact Lens Company made were called the microlens. The design was relatively simple, with the single CN bevel. Plastic rods made of PMMA were cut into buttons. The buttons were placed on machine lathes to cut the interior and exterior radii of curvature, beveled and polished. These lenses were not the most comfortable to wear because of lid irritation. Patients often had a characteristic upheld head to minimize the irritation of the lenses on the lids. The head-tilted-back position and watery eyes gazing down at you was a clue that the person was wearing contact lenses.

Newton wrote, "All contact lenses prior to 1954 for the most

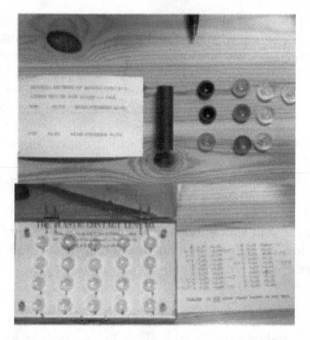

1946 PMMA rods and slugs with PCL microlens trial fitting set. (Roy Wesley personal collection)

part distorted the cornea, whether it was the old fluid lenses or the micro lenses, which were developed in Germany by Wilhelm Soehnges, Frank Dickinson and Dr. Jack Neil of Philadelphia in the early 1950s."

The lenses were fitted so flat that they altered the corneal layer, but inadvertently helped the nearsighted patient by changing the shape in a positive way. He continued:

> We worked very hard to create the Sphercon Lens, a lens that Dr. Jessen and I thought we could recommend that did not distort the eye, fitted on a layer of tears, following the curvature of the eye, and a tear pump was formed in the center. The Sphercon Lens used the natural pumping action of the lids to exchange fluid under the lens, and developed a tear reservoir in the periphery of the lens with an alignment fit between the center of the eye and the periphery. The lenses were made smaller, thinner, and lighter than all

previous ones. We applied for a patent in the United States, Canada, Japan, Britain, and other countries. I believe all the patents were granted except in the United States where the patent still lies in the patent office—there were so many technicalities involved.

We created lenses that were called Tri-curve lenses for keratoconus patients, and we began to realize these lenses helped to hold the original shape of the cornea—in other words, they would not cause distortion—and one could go from contact lenses to spectacle lenses without altering vision. Up to this point, I was never at ease with contact lenses even though we had not had true adverse reactions with the various lenses. (Wesley, 1988, p. 68)

Instruments for Contact Lenses

Simultaneous with the production of reliable contact lenses was the need for precision measurements of the lenses. The optics of the lenses could be determined easily using spectacle lens lensometers (optical instruments to verify a prescription) already in use and adapted to the smaller size of the contact lens. New instrumentation was needed to precisely calibrate, measure, and standardize other unique lens parameters such as the diameter, the inner and outer curvatures, and bevels. Newton collaborated with Sam Mattie (George Samuel Mattie) in 1958 to form a company initially called Plascon Products and re-named Plasmatic, Inc. located on Mannheim Road in Des Plaines, Illinois. Mattie was an optical engineer specialist who invented and manufactured devices that fit the requirements of the time in his tool and die factory.

Some of the early devices produced were instruments to measure the contact lens diameter in millimeters with an accuracy to 0.1mm and lens thickness gauges, accurate to 0.01mm. Calibration tools were produced that were named "contactometers" to standardize convex and concave surfaces on keratometers or ophthalmometers. As doctors began to polish and modify contact lenses in their office, the automatic lens edgers and polishers were manufactured and sold along with adjustment kits. Eventually, Wesley-Jessen produced catalogs with over 250 contact lens related products to support the contact lens market (WJ 1971 Product Catalog).

8 DEVELOPMENT OF WESLEY-JESSEN

Newton was an energetic man with a positive outlook. He looked for opportunities to fulfill his goals in the best possible way. These characteristics helped Newton Wesley build an American business during the 1950s corporate expansion period. In searching for solutions to problems in making a precision contact lens in a reproducible fashion, Newton used all available resources at the time. Newton had an instinct for quickly sizing up people, and he had an innate curiosity about people that tried to understand how people got to where they were in life. He was charismatic and used his charm to make a person feel like they had a new best friend in a matter of minutes. It didn't matter if the person were a waiter, elevator man, or CEO of a company.

He met Paul Smythe through mutual friends early upon his arrival in Chicago. Paul Smythe was the jukebox king, with thirty jukebox patents. Paul invited Newton to participate in an investment in the Kolograph Corporation, which made 16-mm projectors in Indianapolis, Indiana. There was no apparent connection between the manufacturing of film projectors with producing contact lenses. Newton often thought beyond the ordinary to attempt something that others did not see. Although hesitant, he agreed to invest because he thought there might be a possibility of improving contact lens manufacturing through precision engineering. The projector was a diversion and not a good model for making contact lenses, but the engineering concepts helped develop a gauge for measuring the lens diameter. Another development was the WJ Contactometer, which could measure the curve of the contact lens.

Paul Smythe was a colorful man whose flamboyant life landed him in the Chicago newspapers when he was divorcing his first wife. An article in the *Chicago Tribune*, February 23, 1945, reported that Paul Smythe was in a court battle with his ex-wife. It described him as a jukebox maker who was a former bricklayer. His wife wanted funds from the investment she made in his first jukebox patent. His

Paul Smyth Changer and the Rock-Ola Model A Jukebox was issued Patent No. 2,159,832. Newton was captivated by this charming and engaging hustler. He wrote about Paul saying:

> He had about thirty patent rights on the jukebox and worked with Rockola, Seeburg and other companies in the field. I remembered when I was going to high school and college how I could not get over the mechanism of the jukebox. I often wondered what kind of a man was involved with the jukebox. I watched Paul Smythe buy and sell buildings and develop the American Motor Scooter Company. He would often ask me to participate, but I declined, saying it was not in my interest. (Wesley, 1988, p. 62)

Newton might have been financially better off investing in the other ventures instead of Kolograph, which he purchased, changed the name to National Sound Projector Corporation in 1949, and finally filed for bankruptcy on May 27, 1954. Newton learned a lesson from the investment that had only one contact lens manufacturing application. A few years later, he had an opportunity to invest in a new development for a building across the street from his offices, the Mid-Continental Building at 55 East Monroe. He declined the offer saying, "I only invest in things related to the contact lens business. It's the only thing I really know." Had he invested, it would have paid off handsomely. Even so, he never regretted living by his principle.

When Newton was negotiating with Paul Smythe on Kolograph, he relied on Irwin Panter, a Chicago attorney. Irwin became one of his best friends and an advisor and confidant to him in business deals. Newton, Irwin, and Dave Coustan, an accountant, took a four-hour train ride to Indianapolis to discuss the Kolograph Corporation deal. Irwin Panter and Newton developed a deep and lifelong relationship that began in those days of 1945. Irwin was the opposite of Newton in personality: quiet, introspective, thoughtful, and intelligent. Irwin Panter and his legal firm handled many legal battles and corporate administrative documents over the years. As often happened with Newton and his business associates, their lives merged in the social and family spheres, and Irwin's family became a part of Newton's family.

Developing a Market

The term "contact lens" did not appear in *Webster's Dictionary* until 1945. It appeared in the "New Words" section at the back of the 1945 edition of *Webster's New International Dictionary*. References to the "first contact lens" in earlier conjectures on its origin are anachronisms, placing a current term for a concept that had not been so designated. Thus, we repeatedly read that "in 1508, Leonardo Da Vinci created the first contact lens." He did not. He illustrated a man's head in a glass bowl of water with optical lines of reference showing a refraction effect to the back of the eye. One might infer from this drawing that this could be interpreted as a fundamental principle for a future contact lens. This inference would be historical revisionism. In any case, public knowledge of contact lenses from 1940 to 1950 was almost non-existent. In a world devoid of contact lenses, Dr. Wesley brought the concept and product to doctors and their patients. Newton was fond of saying that "the National Eye Research Foundation (NERF) put the words 'contact lens' in the dictionary"; the fact is that the words existed in the dictionary (1945) before he created NERF (1956). Newton and NERF did popularize contact lenses to the extent that the term became common household words.

Training Doctors of Optometry

Newton Wesley was a natural-born teacher. Newton's experience training optometrists at North Pacific College of Optometry, Monroe College of Optometry, and giving post-graduate courses at the American Optometric Center prepared him to continue teaching doctors in fitting contact lenses. He was inquisitive and passionate about understanding how eyes worked and how to improve vision. The business of contact lenses became a challenge when he realized that education and training were necessary to sell the contact lenses his company was producing. He needed to reach out and train core groups of licensed doctors and opticians who would fit the public. Contact lenses were so new as a product in the market that there were no courses in the schools of optometry or ophthalmology to train the eye doctors. In the beginning, Newton spoke to doctors individually or in small classes about contact lenses.

When a doctor or optician expressed an interest in the possibility of fitting contact lenses, Newton would schedule an appointment to demonstrate, train, and provide information about building a contact lens practice. A specialty practice was a novel concept then. On weekends or during summer vacations, doctors who lived in surrounding states like Wisconsin, Michigan, Indiana, or Iowa would receive a personal visit accompanied by his family. It was an opportunity to take his wife and two boys on a road trip out of the city. These drives out to eye doctors helped to persuade doctors to begin fitting the contact lenses that Newton's company was making. He started by building his customer base one by one. The outreach slowly expanded to giving seminar presentations on fitting lenses to groups of doctors, opticians, and technicians in various cities.

His teaching and training schedule increased to the point that Newton decided to learn to fly a plane to reach doctors in smaller communities. Commercial airlines did not fly into small communities of 25,000 people where the average optometrist practiced. Commercial airlines in the 1950s were flying DC-3 and DC-6 planes. Jet planes were not available until October 1958 when Pan American introduced overseas flights on Boeing 707s. Newton said the following to explain why he decided to take up flying:

One night I had finished a lecture at eleven o'clock on a Friday night, and I wanted to get home. I could not get a direct flight from Birmingham to Chicago. I had to backtrack to Atlanta and I waited from 2:00 P.M. to 5:00 or 6:00 A.M. before I could get a flight out. I thought there must be an easier way. Shortly afterwards, I was driving from Chicago to Pittsburgh and I passed through Cleveland—it was a hot summer day, and we did not have air conditioning in the cars as frequently as we do now. I spent the next two hours trying to get through Cleveland, and that did it. I decided to try flying my own plane, and I was scared of flying. I used to be one of those white-knuckle boys, and I remember landing in Washington, D.C. in a dense fog and really, the birds were walking. I could not figure out how the pilot ever found the airport. I was never at ease in a plane, but to get my work done, it had to be, so I took up flying. (Wesley, 1988, p. 80)

Newton began taking flying lessons at Ravenswood Airport on Touhy Avenue near Rosemont, IL. The airport opened during the late 1920s and closed in the early 1960s, the victim of a nearby highway and O'Hare airport expansions. During its operating days, Ravenswood trained many pilots on the GI Bill and later private citizens like Newton Wesley. During Newton's training period, he would have flying nightmares and awaken in a sweat, screaming and thrashing in bed. Nonetheless, he persisted in his flying lessons. Once Newton set a goal for himself, he was tenacious in seeing it through to the end, no matter the consequences.

Newton reached his goal of getting his license to fly and kept up the required number of flying hours to maintain his license. Through the company, he bought a succession of planes: a single-engine Navion, a single-engine Beechcraft Bonanza, and a twin-engine Beechcraft Model 18, which required two pilots. He hired Vernon J. Fish as his pilot, and he acted as co-pilot for the twin-engine Beech. There were some occasions when Newton would take the family on his flights to his seminars. His son Roy remembers flying with him when he had to go to Denver.

> *He let me sit in the co-pilot seat of the twin Beech to experience the thrill of being upfront in the cockpit with the view of the sky, clouds, and earth below. There were so many dials and levers to watch as the plane, constantly in motion, moved on its guided path. I was instructed to watch essential dials: the altimeter, the compass, airspeed indicator, guides to engine performance (RPM and manifold pressure), oil, and fuel. It was daunting but exciting to be in control of a machine flying through the sky.* (Roy Wesley, personal recollection)

His private plane allowed Newton to fly into smaller airports in cities and regions not serviced by the major corporate airlines. At some point in the 1960s, the insurance company providing the corporate Key Man Insurance policy requested that Newton not fly his private plane. In the event of Newton's death, the insurance company would pay WJ a million dollars. Private planes were risky, and so the insurers required him to fly commercial flights only.

By 1950, he was giving seminars across the country, renting

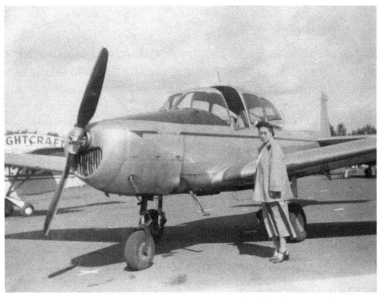

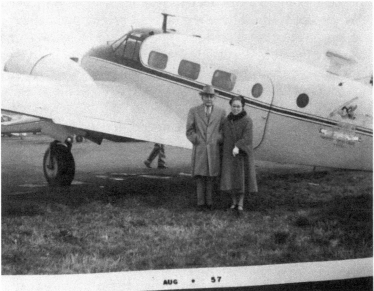

TOP: Dr. Wesley's mother with his Ryan Navion plane, c. 1955. BOTTOM: Dr. Wesley's Beechcraft Model 18 ("Twin Beech" plane, August 1957 with his parents, Portland, Oregon). (Roy Wesley personal collection)

hotel rooms, and presenting his fitting techniques to larger groups. In 1953 he and George published a book, *Contact Lens Practice*, as a guide to fitting contact lenses for professionals. He describes his intent in the foreword, "This book was written with the purpose of acquainting practitioners with simple step by step procedures in fitting the different types of contact lenses." The slim book introduced contact lenses to neophyte doctors and appears primitive by today's standards. Still, it was the beginning of understanding patient selection, optics, ordering specifications of lenses, and fitting them to the doctors of the time.

Dr. Wesley spent many months every year during the 1950s giving courses on contact lens fitting to doctors across the country and the world. These trips also included public relations in each of the cities where he gave classes. He would give radio and television interviews to enhance public awareness of contact lenses. (As an example, the next page shows Dr. Wesley and his staff's schedule for four months in 1955).

Up to this point, the contact lens training courses were teaching methods related to the Microlens, a rigid polymethylmethacrylate lens, before the company introduced the Sphercon lens. The company was transitioning from the Plastic Contact Lens Company to Wesley-Jessen, following the trend to simplify corporate names. Following industry leaders like General Electric (GE), and International Business Machines (IBM), Newton introduced PCL and WJ acronyms. This demanding schedule of courses was in addition to Dr. Wesley's role as president of WJ, requiring administrative, planning decisions, and public relations work. Staffing at WJ was critical to the company's success during this and following periods of growth.

Wesley-Jessen introduced the Sphercon lens in 1956. This innovative lens became widely prescribed in the United States by eye doctors and was well tolerated by their patients. The phenomenal growth in sales doubling every month was a blessing. However, there were growing pains and strains in corporate operations. The popularity and success of the Sphercon lens led to increased exposure and some direct advertising to the public to create more awareness of contact lenses, such as advertisements in *Life Magazine*, one of the most widely distributed and read magazines in the late 1950s. It was also a period of growing prosperity in America, with increased disposable income in most households. Contact lenses were a lux-

THE PLASTIC CONTACT LENS COMPANY

59 EAST MADISON STREET, Suite 417   CHICAGO 2, ILLINOIS

This year we are dividing our courses into two groups. Those of you who have never attended a Wesley-Jessen Microlens Fitting Course should plan to register for this course.

Those of you who have already taken the Wesley-Jessen Microlens Course may attend the post-graduate clinic.

IF YOU HAVE PATIENTS FOR EITHER THE MICROLENS COURSE OR THE POST-GRADUATE CLINIC, PLEASE CONTACT US BEFOREHAND.

You will note that the Post-Graduate Clinic is held in Pittsburgh, Philadelphia, New York and Boston. If it works out in these cities and you like it, we will conduct two separate courses each year in every city.

The Post-Graduate Clinic will cover the latest developments in the contact lens field, and we will cover such specialities as cosmetic contact lens fitting, telescopic contact lens fitting, and keratoconus fitting. We hope to add such things as bevels and cutting lenses later.

FIRST PORTION OF 1955 SPRING SCHEDULE

Dallas, Texas	Sun. Feb. 6	1:00PM-5:00PM	Hotel Adolphus	Micro Cse.
San Antonio, Texas	Wed. Feb. 9	7:00PM-10:00PM	The Gunter Hotel	Micro Cse.
Houston, Texas	Sun. Feb. 13	1:00PM-5:00PM	The Shamrock	Micro Cse.
New Orleans, La.	Wed. Feb. 16	7:00PM-10:00PM	The Roosevelt	Micro Cse.
Memphis, Tenn.	Sun. Feb. 20	1:00PM-5:00PM	Hotel Peabody	Micro Cse.
Los Angeles, Calif.	Sun. Feb. 27	1:00PM-5:00PM	Hotel Statler	Micro Cse.
San Francisco, Calif.	Wed. Mar. 2	7:00PM-10:00PM	St. Francis Hotel	Micro Cse.
Honolulu, Hawaii	Sun. Mar. 6	1:00PM-5:00PM	Royal Hawaiian Hotel	Micro Cse.
Nashville, Tenn.	Sun. Mar. 20	1:00PM-5:00PM	Dinkler-Andrew Jackson	Micro Cse.
Birmingham, Ala.	Mon. Mar. 21	7:00PM-10:00PM	Thomas Jefferson	Micro Cse.
Atlanta, Ga.	Wed. Mar. 23	7:00PM-10:00PM	Atlanta-Biltmore	Micro Cse.
Louisville, Ky.	Tue. Apr. 12	7:00PM-10:00PM	The Brown Hotel	Micro Cse.
Cincinnati, Ohio	Wed. Apr. 13	7:00PM-10:00PM	Netherland-Plaza	Micro Cse.
Dayton, Ohio	Fri. Apr. 15	7:00PM-10:00PM	The Dayton-Biltmore	Micro Cse.
Charleston, W. Va.	Sat. Apr. 16	7:00PM-10:00PM	The Ruffner Hotel	Micro Cse.
Columbus, Ohio	Sun. Apr. 17	1:00PM-5:00PM	The Neil House	Micro Cse.
Akron, Ohio	Thu. Apr. 21	7:00PM-10:00PM	Mayflower Hotel	Micro Cse.
Cleveland, Ohio	Sun. Apr. 24	1:00PM-5:00PM	Hotel Statler	Micro Cse.
Pittsburgh, Pa.	Sun. May 1	1:00PM-5:00PM	Carlton House	Micro Cse.
Pittsburgh, Pa.	Sun. May 1	1:00PM-5:00PM	Carlton House	Post-Graduate Clinic

....

Please enroll me for your no charge Instructional Course to be given in:

I wish to bring a patient to your Clinic for consultation in:

City_____ State_____   City_____ State_____
Date_____ Time_____   Date_____ Time_____

Signed_____   This patient has lenses____.
Address_____   This patient does not have lenses____.
City_____ State_____

Dr. Wesley's February to May 1955 training classes in contact lenses schedule. (Roy Wesley personal collection)

ury item, costing between $150 to $200 a pair (the doctor's fee to patients). Specialty lenses such as toric or bifocal could command even higher prices.

An optometrist reflected in *Contact Lens Spectrum* that "The clinical 'breakthrough' in my practice and the contact lens industry began in April 1956 ... [when] practitioners began fitting Wesley-Jessen's Sphercon corneal lenses" (Goldberg, 2003). The unique features of the Sphercon lens compared with other contact lenses of the day were that it was smaller and centered better on the eye. This resulted from its physical characteristics, with lens diameters ranging from 6 to 9 mm and outer edge bevels that allowed for greater tear flow and comfort.

The Sphercon lens's success was based on the education of the public through the National Eye Research Foundation and the training of eye doctors to fit contact lenses properly. Newton K. Wesley was a driving force in both. The many years of his training doctors across the nation and in other foreign countries paid off in increased awareness and sales of contact lenses in general.

Wesley-Jessen held training sessions to fit Sphercon lenses at branch offices and held regional meetings to extend training and introduce new products to doctors and opticians. The sessions became continuing education courses with accreditation for maintaining state licenses in eye care. Wesley-Jessen held the "First National Contact Lens Congress" in three cities across the United States. The series occurred in November 1956: New York, Chicago, Los Angeles. In January 1957, *Contacto* reported on these meetings. These meetings were more regional than national, but they did lead up to the First World Contact Lens Congress held August 2-4, 1959, at the Edgewater Beach Hotel in Chicago, Illinois.

Creating Public Awareness through Newspapers, Radio, TV

Newton's life had many press-worthy moments that could be turned into headlines. A young graduate of North Pacific University School of Optometry buys school. Twenty-four-year-old President of Portland's Japanese American Citizens League fights for Japanese Americans' freedom during World War II. Optometrist going blind develops a cure through contact lenses. Newspapers articles appeared on each of those subjects and many others during his life.

As he traveled throughout the country giving contact lens training sessions to doctors, Newton had press releases sent out to the local area and offered free local press to the participating doctors if they desired. In time, these efforts generated thousands of newspaper articles per year. Radio and TV stations frequently picked up the releases and interviewed Newton.

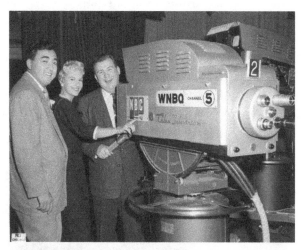

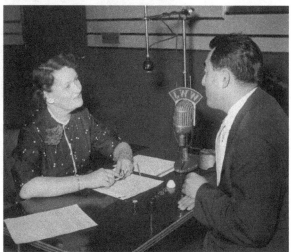

TOP: Dr. Newton K. Wesley on the "Bob & Kay" show, WNBQ (later WMAQ), Chicago, 1959. BOTTOM: Dr. Wesley radio interview on WWJ, Detroit, 1955. (Roy Wesley personal collection)

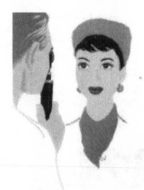

CONTACT LENSES?

only your

family eye doctor

is qualified to

decide

When you purchase contact lenses, consult your eye doctor. Don't risk short-cuts or take chances on so-called bargains when your eyes are involved. Select a reliable doctor and follow his advice. Under his professional care, you will join the millions of Americans who now enjoy normal living through better sight with contact lenses.

FREE!
For additional information, send for booklet: "What is the Cost of Contact Lenses to You?"

**W/J SPHERCON°
CONTACT LENSES**
The world's smallest, lightest and thinnest contact lenses. Worn by more people than any other kind.

"Normal vision with natural good looks"

THE PLASTIC
CONTACT LENS
COMPANY

30 East Madison Street
Chicago 3, Illinois

Trademark

In an unconventional move, WJ placed advertisements in the popular press like *Life* magazine during the late 1950s. Direct-to-consumer advertising by manufacturers was not done at the time because the market was limited. There were no federal regulations at the time. Contact lenses were classified as medical devices by the Food and Drug Administration (FDA) in 1976, but the use of PMMA lenses were grandfathered, so the regulations did not apply.

The eye doctors were the best marketers of contact lenses to the public because by choosing to provide WJ lens-

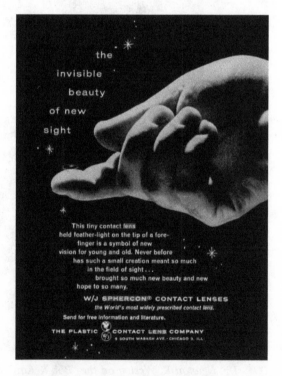

LEFT: Life *magazine, April 28, 1958. RIGHT:* Life *magazine, November 23, 1959.*

es to patients, they furthered the company's growth. The efforts that Newton put into initial training and services to the doctors paid off in product sales. To support doctors in their local areas, WJ's public relations department wrote complimentary press releases for doctors to send to their local newspapers stating that the doctor was attending a seminar or Congress as part of continuing education in the field of contact lenses. The WJ sales staff and national WJ seminars introduced and helped develop new products. NERF, as an outcome of corporate Wesley-Jessen, is discussed in the next chapter.

The inspiration and origin of NERF World Congresses began with Newton Wesley's travels to Europe to attend the International Society of Contact Lens Specialists (ISCLS) meetings sponsored by Wilhelm ("Willy" or "Billy") Söhnges in 1956. The ISCLS was organized in Germany in 1953 based on the initial friendship and meeting of Wilhelm Söhnges and Frank Dickinson at St. Anne's, Lancashire, in 1939 to discuss contact lenses and their design. The American Jack Neill, who was at the nearby Royal Air Force Burtonwood base (a joint UK-US airbase during WWII) joined Söhnges and Dickinson in discussions. The three men created a common goal to develop the micro-corneal lens in 1952. Söhnges converted his Lake Chiemsee (Urfahn am Chiemsee) home into a conference center to house meetings of contact lens specialists in 1955. Söhnge invited Newton to join the ISCLS specialists the following year. Wilhelm Söhnges and Newton Wesley had parallel careers in contact lenses. Both created small corneal lenses, taught, researched locally and internationally, and developed multiple successful organizations. The following year, 1957, Newton and his family were the guests of Willy Söhnges when he attended the ISCLS meetings. Every day the family was transported by motorboat to the adjacent island, Herren Chiemsee. King Ludwig II built a palace on the island in 1878 to resemble Versailles, and the Wesleys had guest rooms nearby. There was an evening chamber music concert in the Great Hall of Mirrors with all the gilt chandeliers lowered from the ceiling and 4,000 candles lighted by hand. The attendees experienced a spectacular sight and sound event. The children of some of the ISCLS participants tended to stay together during the meetings: Muriel "Twinkie" Dickinson, Frank Dickinson's daughter; Robert "Bobbie" Danker, Fred Danker's son; and Lee and Roy Wesley. While the doctors discussed contact lenses, their families enjoyed the Bavarian alps' peace and serenity, the forests, the lake, and the beautiful charm of this region. Frank Dickinson wrote in the October 1957 *Optician*:

> Dr. Newton K. Wesley contributed a valuable statistical report on the comparative results of microlens fitting and "Sphercon" lenses. This new type of lens is smaller than the microlens (from 7mm to 9.2mm in diameter) and is located apically, with a limited amount of free movement over the corneal surface. Dr. Wesley went on to refer to the aims and objects of the Eye Research Foundation.... (Dickinson, 1957, p. 302.)

The ISCLS meeting was a taste of what international conferences could offer. Newton was charmed by the experience and hoped to provide similar experiences for doctors in America. The collegiality and sharing of information were a definite draw for Newton and the others. They were able to see that their families enjoyed themselves as well.

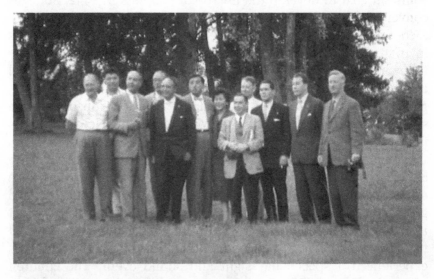

International Society of Contact Lens Specialists, Urfarn, Germany. Robert Danker, Fred Danker, Frank Dickinson, John C. Neill, Willy Söhnges, Newton Wesley, Cecilia Wesley, Erwin Voss, Clifford Hall, Henri Biri, K. Clifford Hall. Söhnges' estate, Urfahn, Bavaria, 1957. (Roy Wesley personal collection)

Dr. Söhnges created the Herschel Gold Medal to honor exceptional contact lens specialists in recognition of outstanding original contributions to contact lens design techniques and of fitting and application in clinical practice. The medal also honored educators and those advancing the practice of contact lenses. Gold medals were also awarded for valuable contributions to the science of contact lenses by those outside the ophthalmic profession. Sir Frederick William Herschel was known for his work in astronomy in the discovery of Uranus, and his son, Sir John Herschel, whose interest in optics and astronomy helped in understanding astigmatism caused by the cornea.

According to the ISCLS, Newton K. Wesley, co-founder of Wesley-Jessen, is the only person to have been awarded the medal twice. He received the award in 1969 and again in 1993. George Jessen was an early Herschel recipient in 1964.

The 1957 family excursion to Europe visited popular cities during which Newton met with contact lens specialists in each location. For example, among those he met were Norman Bier, Robert Fletcher, Clifford Hall in London; Pierre Lemoine, Peter Yven, in Paris. Robert Fletcher and Norman Bier were early pioneers in fitting scleral contact lenses in London and influential specialists during their lifetimes.

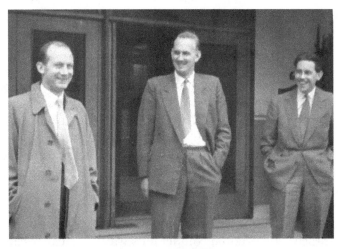

Robert Fletcher, Mr. Dunn, Norman Bier, London, England, 1957 meeting with Newton Wesley. (Roy Wesley personal collection)

85

Newton met with the ophthalmologist Professor Dr. H. J.M. Weve from Utrecht before flying to Kiel, Germany, while his family toured Amsterdam. In Kiel, Newton met with Adolf Wilhelm Müller, a descendant of Adolf Alvin Müller, who gave him an original glass-blown scleral lens made in 1887. The scleral lens Newton obtained was important because it was the same year that Dr. Sämisch of Bonn ordered a glass shell from the prosthetic eye maker Friedrich A. Müller of Wiesbaden to successfully fit a keratoconic patient for the first time. The glassblowers made a modified prosthetic eye with a clear glass central area for vision. These 1887 lenses preceded the publication of articles using various German terms for the device: *Kontackt-Schale*, (F.A. Müller, 1887) *Kontaktgläser* (Anton Müller, 1888), *Hornhautlinsen* (August Müller, 1889) and *"Contactbrille"* (Fick, 1892). English translations: contact shell, contact glasses, corneal-lenses, and contact spectacles, respectively. Karl Otto Himmler made glass scleral lenses for August Müller and Eugène Fick. Müller reported in 1889 that he corrected his -14.00D myopia with a glass shell made by Himmler. R.M. Pearson's research into Himmler's unique contribution concluded:

> Karl Otto Himmler merits wide recognition as the first manufacturer of a contact lens for which the dimensions and power had been specified by the medical student, August Müller. The lenses that he made were a glass, preformed scleral design and had been ground and polished. Nearly a century after they had been manufactured, they were considered to have been well made. (Pearson, 2007, p. 15)

The historical importance of the 1887 contact lens Newton brought home from Kiel was the impetus for the 100th Anniversary edition of the 1987 *Contact Lens Spectrum*. Other publications, (e.g., *Survey of Ophthalmology*, 1989) have chosen to celebrate 1889 as the origin of contact lens history with the publication of August Müller's dissertation on correcting his vision with the Himmler lens made to Müller's specifications.

Newton had a mold made of the Wiesbaden lens and distributed 100 copies of the reproduced lens on a plastic stand as an anniversary remembrance. The original contact lens was not clear because lead was incorporated into the glass, giving the lens a dark appearance. The reason for the additive is unknown.

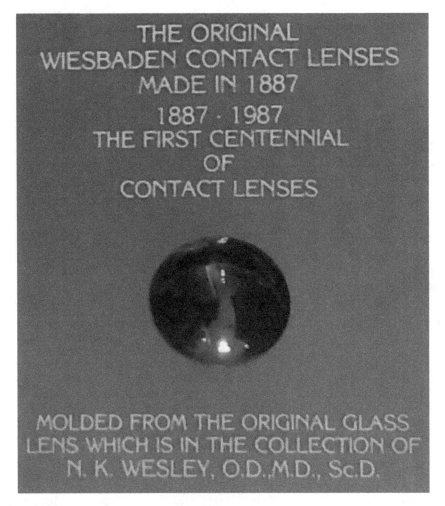

Replica of 1887 Wiesbaden scleral lens from Adolf Müller given to Newton Wesley in Kiel, Germany, 1957. (Roy Wesley personal collection)

The Lab

Manufacturing contact lenses was at the heart of Wesley-Jessen's business. Ever since February 13, 1946, when Newton moved the crude lens-making operation from the Kenmore Avenue basement to the Mallers Building, he considered that date the beginning of the Plastic Contact Lens Company. The all-consuming task of making a small effective contact lens took two years of devoted work. Newton wrote, "We worked Saturdays after the practice, evenings, nights, Christmas, New Year's, and all the other holidays trying to make plastic contact lenses" (Wesley, 1988, p. 58).

A second-hand industrial Briggs and Stratton lathe replaced the home-made foot pedal sewing machine when the basement research operation moved downtown. The lathe was modified to cut the inside and outside curves of plastic buttons to make contacts. The industry's growth led to leasing the entire 9th floor of the Champlain Building (37 South Wabash in 1958) to manufacture contact lenses. From the 1944 experiments to make contact lenses, to the move to the Mallers Building, and then to the Champlain Building, manufacturing took place in what was called "The Lab" because production procedures were also being researched, refined, and developed.

The first employees of the company, outside of the founders, were hired in the production of the lenses: Charles "Chuck" Nishimura; an engineer, James Kawabata; and Joseph Cinefro, who went on to become the lab supervisor and eventually vice-president of NERF.

During the critical years of Wesley-Jessen's development, Joseph Cinefro was the head of the contact lens manufacturing department. He was a stocky, hearty, no-nonsense man—a commanding figure who ran an orderly and efficient department. He was a smoker, as many were in those days, who occasionally liked to chomp on large fat cigars. He could swear a blue streak that made the object of his scorn wither. He was also a totally compassionate, good-hearted soul and dedicated family man. He and his wife Bobbe (Balbina Cinefro, née Gentile) would often treat the Wesley family, company employees, and clients to a multi-course Italian dinner at their Maywood home. Meals at the Cinefro family featured a table groaning with Italian specialties from fried peppers and sausages, spaghetti with meatballs, and eggplant parmesan that Bobbie would prepare in her kitchen. Tiramisu often completed the repast. Eating in moderation was not allowed. Overlooking the family dining room table above on a china cabinet was the ever-present Santa Lucia, the patron saint of vision, holding a plate with two eyeballs on it. The devotion to eye care and their work was omnipresent.

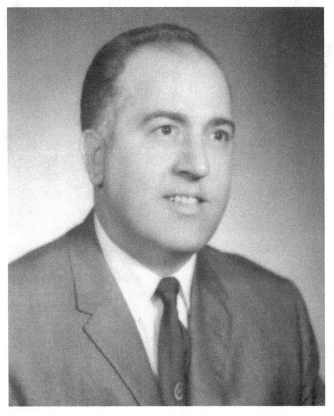

Joseph Cinefro, 1921-1977. (Roy Wesley personal collection)

The three Wesley-Jessen company leaders—George, Newton, and Joe—became recognized in the industry for their dedication and contributions. For example, the Contact Lens Manufacturers Association (CLMA) awarded the Dr. Joseph Dallos Award to Newton Wesley in 1976, George Jessen in 1976, and Joseph Cinefro in 1978. These three men represented the triumvirate of contact lens manufacturing and were deservedly recognized. The Joseph Dallos Award, named after the Hungarian-British contact lens pioneer, is the highest award given each year by the Contact Lens Manufacturers of America "for outstanding contribution to the development and advancement of the contact lens industry and for service to humanity."

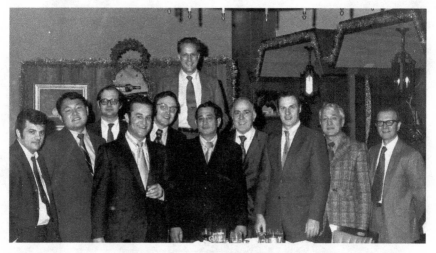

December 10, 1971, WJ Contact Lens Manufacturing staff (left to right): Nick Stoyan, Lee Wesley, Mr. Balinsky, John Panozzo, Charlie Parker, Ralph Kaspari (highest person), Art Pastorello, Joe Cinefro, Kurt Wehking, Jimmy Pastorello, Steve Kondos. (Roy Wesley personal collection)

Some Wesley-Jessen employees started work in "The Lab" and went on to develop their own contact lens companies, making significant contributions in the industry, e.g., Nick Stoyan (Contex), Kurt Wehking, Boyd Richardson (GP Contact Lens), and others. Leonard Bronstein, the editor of *Contacto* magazine for NERF, developed novel designs for gas permeable lenses and bifocals. Bronstein also did significant work on keratoconus. The Arizona Optometric Association sponsors an annual "Bronstein Contact Lens & Cornea Seminar" in his honor. The American Academy of Optometry Founders' Award has been presented to many doctors whose career was touched by Newton Wesley: Alan Tomlinson, Patrick Caroline, Craig Norman, Nick Stoyan, John DeCarle, Robert Morrison, and Joseph Golberg. Many prominent international contact lens fitters were trained or associated with Newton Wesley: Hikaru Hamano, Japan; Victor Chiquiar-Arias, Mexico; Erwin Voss, Argentina; and many more.

Eye Research Foundation and the National Eye Research Foundation (NERF)

Newton incorporated the Eye Research Foundation on October 10, 1956. A non-profit component (The Fund of the National Eye Research Foundation) was incorporated three years later on July 6, 1959. Dr. Wesley created NERF as a non-profit education provider on contact lenses to doctors and the public. NERF provided continuing education seminars to the profession and disseminated contact lens education articles to the public through local and national media. Newton hired Pat Morrisey to do public relations, and she worked closely with him developing concepts and practices. Newton described the achievements of this outreach:

> In 1959 three national encyclopedias, including the *World Book* and *Encyclopedia Britannica*, included contact lenses in their descriptive literature. It took five years of tremendous effort, fourteen staff members working on nothing but contact lens and eye care stories, and countless radio television, and newspaper interviews, but the words contact lenses went into the English language: A far cry from 'What's contact lenses, Doc?' when I would try to explain them to a patient before that time. (Wesley, 1988, p. 98)

The ability to have Hollywood stars, sports figures, and other prominent people wearing contact lenses was critical in creating an allure and incentive for average Americans to wear contact lenses. Newton wrote of meeting the comedian Phyllis Diller, whom he enlisted to serve on the board of directors for NERF:

> We met quite by accident. I was at the Palmer House in Chicago having lunch and Fritz, the maître d', asked me to talk to Ms. Diller because she was having problems with her contact lenses. So I did and worked with her on her problem. It was amazing how people gathered around at the office to see her. The whispering in the office and the building was that Phyllis Diller was there—word seemed to get out. When we would walk down the street, people would whisper or somebody would say, 'Hello, Phyllis,' and she would wave back. She loved the adoration. I have seen that happen with many others, whether it was Wayne Newton, whose wife was a patient, or the Chicago Bears, who also had the charisma. Our practice examined their eyes and also many of the team management, including George Halas and his son. (Wesley, 1988, p. 107)

As an example of a small world phenomenon during this time, Newton's son, Roy Wesley, was attending college at Washington University and became acquainted with Phyllis Diller's son, Peter Diller, who was enrolled there. Peter Diller left college before graduating to pursue a musical career in Los Angeles. Roy and Peter were unaware of their parents' meeting and work together at the time. Phyllis Diller appeared at NERF meetings on occasion and even brought contact lenses into her comedy routine. Speaking of being in public and ignored (a situation that seldom happened), she quipped,

> It's easy. I just take off the makeup and wig and wear glasses instead of contact lenses. No one knows who I am. So instead of people staring at me, I can stare at them. (Lloyd, 1993)

Newton and George became associated with entertainment and sports personalities as patients.

Pat Morrisey and her public relations staff were instrumental in developing movie star and athlete relationships into stories for the public. An 1959 *Chicago American* article stated that "She [Pat] is as tall, slender, and attractive as any model. She has a wide mouth and a bear-trap mind." The author described her work with Wesley-Jessen:

> Pat could have gone with Proctor Gamble. She chose to work for a firm which seemed headed for quick failure or quick success. She said: "The Plastic Contact Lens company could have gone either way, depending on the thinking that went into it at the time. That's what made it attractive." For two weeks, Pat worked in a library. She studied her product and its field. Her boss - an 18 hour a day man - thought she was loafing. The boss demanded she drop everything and accompany him to Dallas, Houston, and San Antonio as a press agent. She went, unwillingly. She told me: "I worked like a Trojan. I set him up 40 interviews in four days in each town. Afterwards he was nearly dead. He's given me my head ever since." Pat was convinced she could do more for her firm than act as a press agent, setting up news interviews. She had big ideas. She said: "Four years ago, our firm employed 39. Now it employs 460. Then, just 1 million Americans wore contact lenses; now, it's 5 million. My work helped." Each Christmas Pat sits down with her bosses and gives them a prospectus of what she hopes to accomplish in the coming year. She said: "They've never said 'No.' My expense accounts have never been questioned. My raises have been frequent and substantial. I now have my own staff." See why the Publicity club voted Pat Morrisey "best of the year"? It is that loyalty and dedication to their work and to the company that exemplified many of the workers at Wesley-Jessen and helped to grow the company and make it a success. (Murray, 1959)

Pat became the director of Public Relations and headed a staff of 14 people. Among the national television interviews that she helped to arrange were appearances of Newton with the contact lens research rabbit on the "Dave Garroway Show" (1953-1954), the "Steve Allen Show" (1956-1964) and many other local stations and newspaper articles. The rabbit was named "Leo" (after Leonardo Da Vinci) and was fitted with contact lenses to demonstrate the safety and efficacy of contact lens wear to the public. Leo appeared with Newton on the Dave Garroway Show and the Steve Allen Show in 1959. Pat and her team created the idea for having a beauty contest for the First World Contact Lens Congress with designers creating various wearable items for men and women highlighting contact lenses.

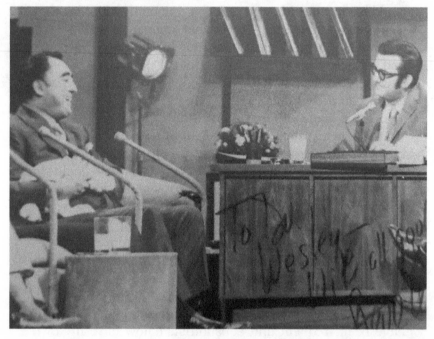

Dr. Newton K. Wesley (left, with Leo the Rabbit by his side) on the Steve Allen Show. February 1971. (Roy Wesley personal collection)

A WJ memorandum from Dr. Newton K. Wesley dated June 14, 1970, directed to "The Planning Committee," expressed his thoughts on objectives and long-range planning. Concerning "Public Relations," he wrote:

> *This has been another area that W/J has tried to help. In the formative contact lens years 1955-1959, W/J spent $500,000 a year for five years to place the words "contact lenses" into the English language. The 2 ½ million dollars that were spent W/J believes has proven its worth in that*

contact lenses have brought an increased fee of at least one hundred million dollars annually in the past 10 years, according to estimates, and it may be higher since there are many others allied to the fitting of contact lenses. Even today, Dr. Wesley writes a column for newspapers and 250 TV and 1200 radio stations use his words on eye care. (Wesley, 1970)

As mentioned before, Newton often told people that WJ and NERF brought the words "contact lens" into the *Merriam-Webster Dictionary*. The compound word "contact lens" made its appearance in the American English language in 1945, when *Webster's New International Dictionary* listed the term in the "New Words" addendum. Newton's description in the memorandum is more accurate for WJ and NERF's role in promoting contact lenses.

The Computer Age

Newton believed that the company was the first to bring computers into the ophthalmic field. In 1958, Newton flew his plane, accompanied by his pilot, Verne Fish, and his secretary, Jan Janies, to White Plains, NY, to attend the International Business Machines (IBM) executive training courses in Endicott, NY. Newton saw the potential of IBM computers for Wesley-Jessen, and he initiated the company's purchase of its first IBM system. The card punch panel, card sorter, and IBM 405 electric punched card accounting machine transformed the company's manually based operations world. It took time for everyone to learn, accept, and adopt new procedures. The next several years saw rapid expansion into the IBM/350 System housed in a dedicated air-conditioned room, as required by the large computers with sorting cards in the 1960s. Newton was surprised at the reaction of some doctors when they were assigned an account number. These doctors felt they lost the personal connection and just became a number. A few went as far as to drop their accounts. Computerization over the years helped the company produce lenses more accurately in addition to streamlining inventory and accounting.

Installation of the IBM 350 system required renting another floor of the Champlain Building at 37 S. Wabash, maximizing the

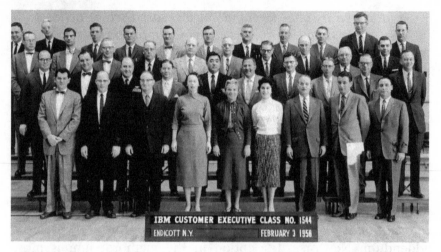

IBM CUSTOMER EXECUTIVE CLASS NO. 1544
ENDICOTT N.Y.   FEBRUARY 3 1958

1959 IBM Executive Training Class. Dr. Newton K. Wesley is in the middle of the second row (5th from the left), and Jan Janies (4th from the right) first row. (Roy Wesley personal collection)

air-conditioning system, hiring staff, and laying out the card punch machines with their operators, card sorter machines, and mainframe units with reels of tapes. Quiet, tall, thin, eyeglass-framed James "Jimmy" Soukup was the man in charge of IBM operations.

IBM was the corporate automation leader. IBM started from multiple companies providing worker time clocks to data tabulations. The companies were consolidated and re-focused to produce computers used by much of the business world. IBM provided hardware and software that kept the nation's businesses moving forward. America's secretarial force typed on IBM typewriters and the rapid, smooth IBM Selectric, with its rotating center ball. An early entry into airline reservations systems was provided by IBM collaborating with American Airlines in developing SABRE (Semi-Automatic Business Research Environment), the first online reservation system for the industry. GE (General Electric) and GM (General Motors) dominated the consumer markets with their ubiquitous products from toasters to cars. The ornate buildings and offices of the General Motors Building (Cadillac Place) and the Fisher Building seemed to be permanent testaments to these corporations' power. IBM, GE, Fisher, and GM did not heed the winds of change or react quickly enough to adapt, resulting in their downfalls. Indeed, Wesley-Jessen did not quickly adapt to the changing market of soft lenses and rigid gas permeable lens chemistry later in its corporate life. Nonetheless, the computerization of Wesley-Jessen led to new developments at the company in billing, sales, accounting, and research.

Surviving Crises

Newton had a resilience born of learning survival skills in Oregon's wild forests, coming of age during the Great Depression, and pulling through incarceration as an innocent Japanese American during World War II. His ability to adapt and thrive during these extraordinary periods of stress was a strength he needed during the unfolding dilemmas encountered during Wesley-Jessen's expansion.

There was a period of rapid growth for five years from 1950 to 1955 in the contact lens field in the United States and Wesley-Jessen was the foremost leader in that period. Many new contact lens manufacturers entered the market to imitate WJ's success and to take market share. The company became a desirable target for a buyout from American Optical (AO), the largest American optical company (mostly spectacles at the time), with approximately 450 branches. Wesley-Jessen seriously considered the offer over a two-year evaluation period. The terms would have been an exchange of AO stock valued at $2.5 million with an estimated eventual value of $5 to $6 million to take over WJ. Newton and George decided to turn it down because "we would rather paddle our own canoe." Nonetheless, the issue of growing the business required an infusion of capital.

In the world of investment banking, mergers, and acquisitions, then as today, there are no friends or emotions. Decisions were made based on profit production either immediately or in the future. Newton was caught in a web of intrigue during this period of growth. He and WJ were vulnerable because of the need for cash to expand and grow into the future. Newton did not imagine at the time that people could be evil and manipulate a growing business into a hostile takeover situation. Newton described his solution given the need for capital:

> We consulted experts in the field, and it was the consensus not to have a general offering. I only wanted to offer 15 percent

of the total stocks outstanding and that we would, under the SEC laws, be required to have only fifteen investors. Our thought was to raise $1.5 million, which meant fifteen blocks of $100,000 each. Large insurance companies, an individual from a large bank, Texas oil millionaires, two large insurance companies, etc. formed the group. I thought that selling off 15 percent of our stock would be safe, that is, we would not lose control by holding 85 percent of the stock—Dr. Jessen and I being equal partners. So I thought!

The investors were very clever. They picked a leader and a follower (two people) plus the investment bankers to represent them. No sooner had we raised the $1.5 million than the bank called our loan. We argued that the $650,000 loan should have been renewed. In fact, they should have increased our line of credit since we had raised $1.5 million more, but the bank demanded repayment and did pay themselves off. Even as we walked into the meeting completing the deal, and our bank account representative was telling us that we would have a larger line of credit, the bank representative agreed. The investors had wanted two people on the board to represent them, and we had agreed to that request prior to the placement of the $1.5 million issue. The purpose of selling off 15 percent of the stock was to have a greater line of credit for expansion. Later on, we learned that there was a hidden investor in the bank who held a block of $100,000, and he was the one who called the previous loan and left us like a sitting duck for the takeover. (Wesley, 1988, p. 122)

Things went from bad to worse. The investors claimed that the original stock offering was filed on false statements. It took serval months to answer the investors' questions and demands by checking sales, tax records, and manufacturing data to prove otherwise. The process used up valuable time that should have been devoted to manufacturing and growing the business. Suppose there was enough evidence of a false offering. In that case, the investors could and would file a recission suit (contract cancellation) that would demand the total funding to be repaid immediately. The contact lens market had increased in the country, and many new competitors took up market share. Wesley-Jessen began losing $50,000 a month at a time they needed to be increasing their profits. Individual investors presented new problems and demands to be resolved, usually on a Friday afternoon, to increase the pressure and lead the company to collapse.

There seemed to be collusion among the Chicago banks not to back another loan to Wesley-Jessen. Newton had an offer from a long-time friend, Sam Lane, to use his collateral of a million dollars as the basis for getting a loan to cover the outstanding debt. They went to many banks together and were unable to secure more than a $50,000 commitment from any bank, even banks that were friendly to Wesley-Jessen at the company's beginning. Sam Lane was in the 1945 Monroe College graduation class photo with George Jessen at Monroe College of Optometry, when Newton taught there, so they had a long-standing relationship. Newton tried to reciprocate Sam's kindness by helping Sam in his contact lens insurance business when it was in trouble, and later, by placing him on the Pacific College of Optometry board. Sam was also on the NERF board for many years.

With the strength of his personality and character, Newton Wesley was able to find a solution to settling the investor's battle by paying back the entire loan. The idea came to him after a friend and business associate, Evelyn Corral of Contacts, Inc., told him privately,

> I know you are in trouble, and the grapevine says that the investors are trying to take you over. I know you can't talk, but if you need any money, please contact me. I do not have a lot, but whatever I have, I am willing to help. (Wesley, 1988, pp. 137-138)

That conversation set Newton into action, and he called fifteen doctors that he knew well and had worked with to a meeting in Chicago and, after explaining the investors' battle to them, he was able to raise $250,000 from the group. By relying on friends, he finally paid back the investors and kept the company from a takeover. Other associates such as his attorney and friend, Irwin Panter, and others that Newton relied on chipped in what they could to help him out. Many contributors held on to the stocks issued in payment for their help. The increase in their share value when Wesley-Jessen was sold to Schering-Plough helped to repay their generous assistance. At the end of the nearly two year battle with the banks and investors to keep his company, Newton said in response to Irwin Panter's question of how he was doing,

> I'm fine; I'm happy. Even though I am beaten to a pulp, I am learning. ... I don't wish the experience I went through on anyone. All the lights on Wabash Avenue and State Street were lit up like Christmas and, yet, it was broad daylight. The elimination of stress must have relieved my shoulder muscles, the capillaries in my brain and eyes—I could see so much clearer. It was quite a feeling....We had won the investor's battle! (Wesley, 1988, p. 139)

The fight to retain control of the company forced Newton to realize that he needed help managing and creating a profitable future for Wesley-Jessen. Besides emotionally draining pressures of the investors trying to take his company, he had to manage and plan for the company daily, travel nationally and internationally every month to give seminars and training, do public relations, and have some time for his family. The investors did a worldwide search for a president to manage operations at Wesley-Jessen while trying to reduce Newton's share to less than 50% of the company. The investors and Wesley-Jessen board interviewed two of the candidates, but neither was entirely right. After Newton re-gained control of his company, he actively sought professional-managerial help. The first attempts were to find a vice-president/general manager who could be groomed to become the president. It seemed to be working until four years when things fell apart and, Newton realized he needed to use a national recruiting firm to find the right professional fit. It took a year of interviews and planning to select Orrin Stine, who came from Borden Company as chemical division head. Orrin's family had started Stineway Drugstores in Chicago. Orrin became the president overseeing daily operations and planning while Newton was the chairman of the board. Orrin had his work cut out for him since the FDA approved the Wichterle soft lens for sale and distribution in the United States when Orrin was hired to start at Wesley-Jessen.

Labor Union Troubles

The early American labor movement beginning in the mid-19th century was a noble endeavor applying social justice, equality, and fairness for workers. Idealism turned to greed, gangsterism, and corruption by union officials in the 1950s. The Senate McClellan Commission investigated unfair and corrupt labor union practices, resulting in a sweeping housecleaning of the AFL, CIO, and the Teamsters unions. Corruption at the level of top union officials was enforced by strong man tactics at the worker level. Wesley-Jessen was caught up in the labor struggle during this period.

An article appeared in the November 2, 1958, *Chicago Daily Tribune* with the headline "Optical Union Pickets Contact Lens Company," and stated:

> The AFL-CIO United Optical Workers union local 853 began picketing the Plastic Contact Lens Company, 59 E. Madison St., Saturday to seek the right to represent about 200 employes of the company. Lt. Frank O'Sullivan of the police labor detail said 100 employes refused to cross the picket line.

It was not unusual at the time for unions to use intimidation and harassment of employees to influence employees to join the union. Unions infiltrated companies, and carried out espionage of the business and its planning in an attempt to sabotage and force compliance.

Newton was against unionizing the company because he felt that the employees were paid comparable union wages with good fringe benefits (liberal vacations, sick leave, and a profit-sharing plan). Since corporate morale was strong, there was no need to burden employees with additional union dues. His decision was strengthened by an incident that an employee faced, which he described in *Contacts—One Hundred Years Plus*:

> One evening I was working late, and I found one of our women employees crying at the entrance of our building. It was not until I questioned her very carefully that I realized she was afraid. I got the story that she was being roughed up

because her boyfriend was a captain or leader in a possible union takeover in trying to unionize our workers. After I reassured her and helped her outside, I met the union leader as I was about to re-enter the building. He was drunk. As he was talking to me, he sprayed my whole face with the spit that accompanied his alcoholic breath. I thought to myself, 'I am not going to deal with such a union as the Optical Workers in Chicago.' They were part of the Teamsters Union and had only been beaten once. I just did not like their tactics. At the time he was saying that he was going to unionize our shop and wanted to know if I were Dr. Wesley. I nodded my head in the affirmative. It was a very unpleasant meeting. (Wesley, 1988, p. 112)

Another Wesley-Jessen employee was targeted by union organizers and beaten up on his way home after work. The victim came to Dr. Wesley for help and protection. Newton said,

...we hired a private detective specifically to follow this man home and be sure he was not hurt. By labor relations board rules, you cannot do surveillance, but you certainly can protect a worker. For a few nights, the detective carefully followed the worker home and nothing happened. The third night, as the detective was following him, he got waylaid by the worker. The worker thought he was an assailant and the private detective had to tell him why he was there! (Wesley, 1988, 114)

These events and others had a dramatic effect on Newton. He felt personally threatened and he knew that more threats to his employees were possible, so he purchased a handgun for protection that he kept in the top side drawer of his office and during that turbulent time, he even carried it home with him and placed it in the nightstand drawer while sleeping. The move into the new space at 37 South Wabash was to occur at the time the Optical Union was picketing, so Newton decided to delay the move because the Union could interfere and shut down operations for an undetermined length of time. He wrote:

When the union found out that I was not going to move and that I was paying double rent, they hit us with a walkout. Theoretically, we could not have a strike because we were not unionized. During the picketing, there were many threats and people beaten up. One of my employees had a side business, which was totally wrecked. It was not a very pleasant period, but we stuck it out for six weeks, hired a labor attorney, and, on his advice, began to replace workers. Toward the end of the strike, I even had overtures for any type of deal from the union, which, obviously, we would not hear or accept. During this period a sergeant of the police department came in and tried to insinuate that the strike was not over and that the police department could not give us protection. We were not receiving any more protection than normal, but I had to assume that we did have police protecting our workers anywhere, even on the street. There were a number of scuffles on the picket line, and the police would appear like any good police department in the case of a disturbance. One of our men went through the picket line and, in order to defend himself, fought back and pulled a knife. He was wrong for carrying a knife. When he appeared in court, we were fined. The company paid the fine since there was nothing we could do about it. (Wesley, 1988, p. 113)

Regarding his personal fears, Newton wrote:

After the first picket line went up, I remember the first time I got into my car, with I usually parked in a dark alley between buildings at night. It was late, and I actually was afraid to step on my starter. Then I thought, The hell with it. I am not going to be afraid and be scared away. I started the car. I will have to admit I was relieved to still be there. Also, for a doctor to go through the picket lines while we were short of supplies, was no fun, but I drove a truck laden with supplies through the picket lines. (Wesley, 1988, p. 114)

The company moved part of its manufacturing and offices from the Mallers Building at 59 East Madison just down the block to 37 South Wabash, the Champlain Building, under cover of night over a weekend when the union workers would not expect them to move. A north-south alley connected the back of the buildings with access to freight elevators, so the moving company could move furniture and equipment without being detected. This is the same alley that Newton often parked in when he returned to the office late at night and where he described his fear about starting his car during the union picketing. The move was successfully completed without incident.

Wesley-Jessen had some men who were previously members of the Optical Union, such as Newton's partner, George Jessen, who knew the Union president, and Joe Cinefro, the production department's head. There were three Pastorello brothers who all worked for WJ and were former union members. Despite their former union affiliations, none of these workers supported the Optical Union attempts to organize within the company. After the *Chicago Tribune* article appeared about the strike, an Illinois congressman made an appointment to meet with Newton. He said he read the article and was interested in helping small businesses. However, it was clear that the Union sent him when the Congressman tried to persuade Newton to negotiate and settle with the Union. These events coincided with the police sergeant saying he couldn't protect WJ employees against the Union. Despite all this, Newton refused to give in.

In the end, Wesley-Jessen employees voted against joining the Optical Union, and the matter ended without further harassment.

Contact Lens Scare Stories

From the beginning of the introduction of contact lenses as a concept to the public, the press could create interest or public panic about contact lenses. These reports had a direct correlation to company sales and profits. For most of us, it's scary enough to think about putting something into our eyes. When something comes near our eyes as a potential danger, the natural reaction is to blink the eyelids and shut the eyes to prevent harm.

During the 1960s, various scare stories about contact lenses appeared. These articles created an unreasonable fear in some of the public about a sensitive and challenging subject. Newspaper reports circulated claiming that contact lenses made from the chemical methyl methacrylate were toxic and caused blindness. This is true of the liquid chemical form of the molecule. When the liquid is polymerized into the rigid polymethyl methacrylate (PMMA) form, used in the manufacture of hard contact lenses, it is harmless. The later development of soft contact lenses uses a hydrated form, 2-hydroxyethyl methacrylate (HEMA), which has also been found to be safe. Nonetheless, widespread coverage of the chemical causing blindness fueled a debate about the safety of contact lenses that reached the US Senate hearings of 1964, presented by William Stone, Jr., MD, the director of ophthalmic plastic research at the Massachusetts Eye and Ear Infirmary in Boston. He suggested that methyl methacrylate in contact lenses could cause toxic problems leading to infections and blindness. His bottom line was that only ophthalmologists should prescribe contact lenses and not optometrists. Maurice Poster, OD, from New York and the American Optometric Association committee chair on contact lenses and others refuted the claims. The FDA found no evidence for Dr. Stone's claim and vindicated the use and current contact lens fitting practices (Special Committee on Aging, 1964, pp. 413-430).

In the early days, hard contact lens wearers used sterile wetting solutions to clean and make the lenses more comfortable during insertion. The largest provider of wetting solutions was Barnes-Hind. In 1959 there was a bacterial contamination of the wetting solution that prompted a recall by the FDA. The announcement to the press was curious, "Persons who wear contact eyeglasses should avoid using a product called Barnes-Hind Wetting Solution...." The report continued: "FDA scientists have found the product is nonsterile and they have isolated a bacterium, Pseudomonas aeruginosa, in a lot, which can cause blindness" (Departments of Labor, Health, Education, and Welfare, 1961, p. 180).

This statement affected many lens wearers, who stopped buying the product. Newton said that Wesley-Jessen, as a leading buyer of wetting solutions, might have put Barnes-Hind out of business if they asked for their money back on all the stock products. They did not do that, but the public concern was real. Solutions for contact lenses had become a large industry globally, accounting for billions of dollars in sales to support the contact lens industry. They are still subject to contamination problems from time to time.

The wetting solution contamination problem prompted researchers at Wesley-Jessen to develop a potential solution of putting two antimicrobials, hexachlorophene and Corobex®, as effective agents against the known pathogens in the eye, into the contact lens plastic. There was a great deal of push back from the FDA concerning the addition of a chemical into plastic that had the possibility of leaching out. There were forces opposing approval, some of which influenced regulators at the FDA at the time. Arguments to get the patent approved were aided by Dr. Wesley seeking the support of Illinois Senator Everett Dirksen, the minority Senate leader. WJ hired William "Bill" O'Brien to be a public relations person to set up an appointment with Senator Dirksen. Newton described his initial meeting:

> He said, "What can I do for you, Dr. Wesley?" He was very direct and straight to the point, but his eyes twinkled. He tried to put me at ease and was friendly. I told him the whole story of Asptoplast and the FDA. He looked at me and said, "Okay, bring me all the data and set up an appointment with my secretary," which I did. The interview lasted just a few minutes, but I felt that Senator Dirksen was sincere. I liked him.
>
> Five days later, we were back and there was a pile of about four feet of papers on his desk we had sent him. He said, "Okay, I believe you. What do you want me to do? Make it quick, young man, because I will be on the floor in a few minutes." He said, "I'll call over to the FDA right now," and he reached for the phone. I said, "Please Senator Dirksen, do not do that." In mid-air, he stopped his actions and had a surprised look on his face. He turned his head, looked at me quizzically, and asked, "Why not?" I said, "Would you call there and get a speaker for the National Eye Research Foundation, there may be some action from your call." That is exactly what happened. He called over there and asked for a speaker for the National Eye Research Foundation. He explained that two years ago we had applied

for a representative speaker and that we had not received an answer, in spite of repeated requests. He stated that Dr. Wesley was the Chairman of the Board and that Dr. Jessen and I were the founders.

Within a week we had a positive affirmative reply, and it was interesting that Senator Dirksen had told the speaker that he might see him after the meeting because he had an appointment in Chicago.

Senator Dirksen asked me to walk with him to the floor of the Senate. I could feel the power concentrated in this small area, and he was still willing to take time with a small person like me. It made me feel very humble. I do not know what happened internally at the FDA after that. For about two years, we did not hear from the FDA. Oh yes, every once in a while we would hear a rumble, but the pressure was off. I often wonder whether Senator Dirksen just picking up the phone and showing an interest in what was going on with our case was a factor. It did give the FDA time to reconsider the whole matter.

In the end, the FDA stated that we could market the Aseptoplast lens, as we called it. The FDA also stated that we should put on it the legend that this was to be prescribed only by a physician or optometrist. We were very happy because optometrists were able to use contact lenses with a chemical drug in it. It was historic. (Wesley, 1988, pp. 109-111)

It was an historic event because it would be another ten years before Rhode Island passed legislation allowing optometrists to prescribe diagnostic drugs in 1971. Other states followed suit after that. Wesley-Jessen patented the Aseptoplast contact lens in 1964. Also historic was an outcome of Newton's relationship with Senator Dirksen that resulted in Dirksen's speech to Congress honoring Newton Wesley and George Jessen, the contact lens industry, and NERF, which was delivered July 22, 1959. The text of Dirksen's speech was published in the Congressional Record (the document is reproduced in the Appendix).

The People of Wesley-Jessen

Newton Wesley was a people person, as was his partner, George Jessen. They had that natural gift of relating to people, which was probably enhanced early in their career as optometrists engaging in individual patient eye concerns. Newton was a gregarious boss who knew employees on a first-name basis. He greeted not only WJ employees on a first-name basis, but all the people he encountered: car valet men at the underground Grant Park Garage, elevator men, janitors, restaurant maître d's, and waiters. It was not unusual to walk down the street with Newton with someone approaching him, saying, "Hi, Doc! Nice to see you."

Secretaries were essential to Newton's work in managing his daily appointments, meetings, writing correspondence, and making travel arrangements. Some of his secretaries moved on to higher functions within the company. For example, he promoted Jan Janies (Jan's given name was Emma, but preferred to be called Jan Janies) to various positions, including Wesley-Jessen corporation officer (assistant secretary). George Jessen's wife, Lillian Jessen, was officially the corporation secretary, but Jan did the administrative work for the board of directors. Newton used dictation machines and tape recorders for memos, letters, notes, speeches, and other communications that his secretary or the secretarial pool would type in duplicate. Newton carried many pieces of luggage because of his frequent travel schedule, so reducing the weight of his necessary equipment was essential. He was always watching for miniature products in tape recorders, cameras, and other gadgets to simplify his work. His travels to Japan brought him into contact with the latest miniatured business tools, which the Japanese were excellent in manufacturing. Among his many cameras, his favorite was the German-made Minox, which was 3 x 1 x ½ inch thick. When Newton was flying his plane, he had to carry at least two bags for his logbook, navigation charts, flight equipment, checklists, and other items. This was before the advent of roller bags, so he looked like a loaded pack mule. Newton described his luggage dilemma:

> I was carrying so many instruments around that were needed for the courses that I counted something like nineteen pieces of luggage, including 16-mm projectors,

slide projectors, ophthalmometers, supplies, etc., and that was really barnstorming. (Wesley, 1988, p. 79)

Newton had a small staff who helped him organize his equipment and travel needs over the many years he was giving courses.

Being Japanese American, Newton did not have the discriminatory prejudices of hiring only white workers as most downtown companies of the time. He reveled in the diversity of Chicago's population, the transportation system that enabled workers to come into the Loop quickly at a reasonable cost, and the large pool of available workers. He always wanted to keep the company there rather than move out to the suburbs. An early employee was Al Bonhart, an African American. He was a loyal and trusted employee. Al grew with the company over time and became the head of his department until his retirement. Many first-generation Hispanics were hired, mostly in manufacturing, and other areas. Wesley-Jessen was an equal opportunity employer more than a decade before the concept became popularised in the mid-sixties.

Consultation Services

A consultation service was provided to eye care professionals to help problematic lens fitting cases that a doctor had or answer WJ product questions. The consultants were eye doctors who also treated patients in the Wesley-Jessen eye clinic at 37 S. Wabash. They had hands-on experience with the fitting problems that doctors calling into consultation were discussing. Many Illinois College of Optometry students were hired during the summer to assist in handling the consultation calls. Some students became full-time WJ employees after graduation, such as Carole Schwartz, OD, and Jan Jurkus. After their WJ experience, Illinois College of Optometry hired them as faculty. C. Robert Parker, OD, was the Director of Consultation, Chicago Sales Manager, then National Accounts service manager. As the National Accounts manager, Charlie oversaw domestic and overseas accounts. Among the many consultants in the department were Art Hogan, OD, and Brenice Ligman, OD. Many personal relationships developed at WJ, including Art Hogan and his wife, Frances. Co-workers played the role of matchmakers resulting in their 1961 marriage.

Sales Staff

Newton was a one-person traveling salesman when he began training doctors to use company lenses and products. As the optometrists he trained began to have positive results fitting contact lens and increased revenue, other doctors noticed their success and began to learn about contact lenses and fitting. The 1950s were a period of rapid growth for Wesley Jessen, resulting in faster service to doctors and patients with increased profits to WJ. This was accomplished by installing computers and establishing regional branch offices. Some offices had trained optometrists to answer questions for doctors and patients, a sales staff, lab technicians to modify and correct lens specifications on-site, and other education services. At the end of 1959 and the beginning of 1960, 15 United States branch offices were incorporated with several foreign distributors (the Appendix lists branches and distributors).

Wesley-Jessen Research

Newton Wesley began investigating optics and general principles of contact lenses when he realized in 1942 that they could cure his visual affliction caused by keratoconus. Newton would have researched what was known about contact lenses at the Monroe College of Optometry library, where he taught. He may have found William Feinbloom's 1941 articles on contact lenses in the *American Optometric Association Journal*. He later read L. Lester Beacher's *Contact Lens Technique* textbook published in 1941, as evidenced by an edition in his book collection. For the first several years of developing contact lenses, the company had to use "necessity is the mother of invention" as a working principle. Practical needs created the CN bevel, the bonnet system using plastic buttons to cut lenses, polishing, and finishing techniques, to name a few. The initial PMMA used for contact lenses required an understanding of its chemistry, and adjustments in the formulation, curing time and temperature, to produce the best-molded rods for cutting into lenses. In the early 60s, the plastics research moved from the Chicago Loop to an industrial site in Schiller Park with Dr. Homer Hamm, a chemist, in charge of research. Dr. Hamm received his PhD in chemistry from the University of Minnesota. Dr. Hamm investigated cross-linking the PMMA polymers at the industrial park to maintain the bio-inert property necessary to contact lenses, shelf-life stability, and other properties. During his tenure, Dr. Hamm patented a Teflon coating to place on the edges of contact lenses and developed novel plastics, including cellulose acetate butyrate, to promote oxygen transmission through the lens. Dr. Chah Moh Shen and Lee Wesley joined Dr. Hamm as novel cross-linked hydrophilic polymers were developed, leading to the creation of the WJ DuraSoft lens to provide enhanced water content, oxygen transmission, and durability (WJ Patent #4,158,089, June 12, 1979). They were joined later by Dr. Samuel Loshaek as head of the WJ Research department.

Dr. Alan Tomlinson was an optometrist and PhD, DSc from the United Kingdom, who joined the WJ research team and enhanced contact lens research in anterior ocular surface physiology.

Within the research department was an engineering division that included Malcolm Townsley, a mechanical and electrical engineer adept at mathematical calculations, and Malcolm Bibby, an electrical engineer from Liverpool, England, who also held an MBA from the University of Chicago. They were responsible for creating the teamwork behind developing the Photoelectronic Keratoscope (PEK) to map the anterior corneal surface using computer algorithms to determine the best fit for contact lenses. Dr. Wesley used this work as his research dissertation project to obtain his research Medical Degree from Osaka University which he received in 1977. The instrument debuted in 1970, but Newton Wesley conceived of the principle 15 years earlier in 1955. A Polaroid Land Camera was used to take a photo of the cornea overlain by a Placido Disc through the instrument. The Placido Disc is a series of concentric circles that allow the visual interpretation of corneal irregularities such as astigmatism when imaged over the cornea. The image was magnified, and six axial curves were measured on the surface by the computer to generate a topographical map drawn from the numerical data. The curvatures determined the best fit of the lens to the cornea.

Wesley-Jessen Products

Wesley-Jessen offered a full range of eye care instruments and products. There was a time when a new doctor could outfit his

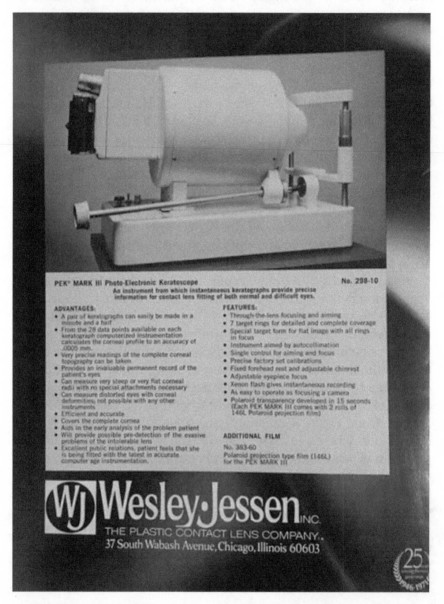

PEK, Photo-Electronic Keratoscope, 1971. (Roy Wesley personal collection)

office with equipment from the WJ catalog: office equipment like examining chairs, phoropters (a device with lenses and dials to determine a patient's vision prescription), keratometers (instrument to measure corneal curvatures), slit lamp biomicroscopes (an intense light tool with a microscope to view the exterior and interior of the eye), and other items. Instruments to measure contact lenses were available such as lensometers for measuring the power of contact lenses, contactogauges for measuring the concave or convex radii of curvature of the contact lenses, Conta-scope for surface and edge inspection of lenses, radiuscopes for checking the base curve of a lens, measuring magnifiers to measure the total lens diameter, Burton lights with ultra-violet black light tubes for checking lens fits and fluorescein staining patterns, thickness gauges to measure the lens thickness at the center or edge and many other devices. Lens adjustment equipment was also sold to doctors who wished to make adjustments on lenses in their office. There were Wesley-Jessen edge polishers, adjustment kits with tools to grind edges of lenses or polish surfaces together with the polishing compounds.

Just four years after the founding of Wesley Jessen, the company manufactured, and sold a new smaller and more comfortable product, the Sphercon lens.

In 1958, Newton successfully applied IBM computers in business routines like accounting, sales, and mailings. He expanded computer applications to the concept that data analysis could be used to aid in the fitting of contact lenses. Later in the 1970s, the Photo-Electronic Keratoscope (PEK) development provided proof that computers had an important role. The computer analysis of corneal data points to calculate a corneal profile gave hope that better fitting lenses would be made with greater comfort. Up to this point in time, contact lenses were cut with a single base curvature, but the natural corneal curvature is not just not one single curve. The new lens designs which could accommodate the computer assisted corneal information appeared as the Autofocal™, Multi-Range®, Asphercon®, and the Dynacurve™, or X-100™ contact lenses. The Autofocal™, Multi-Range®, and Asphercon® lenses were full range vision lenses prescribed for presbyopic patients (those who need assistance in near vision to read or see things more clearly while reading). An increasing plus diopter power add was achieved as the eye looks down with the lens being held in place by the lower eyelid to allow for vision through a lower section of the lens. The Asphercon® lens was developed to follow the cornea's aspheric profile, as determined by the System 2000™ profile. The clinical experience was that the Autofocal lens design offered increased comfort, so the lens design was modified to provide the same comfort for single vision lenses. Therefore modifications for the Dynacurve and Asphercon lenses were made. System 2000 was the name given to the computer print-out of the PEK system's corneal profile. In essence, System 2000 generated more fitting points than would normally be taken by the doctor in taking the usual keratometer reading points. It could also account for irregularities in the mires (images) seen through the keratoscope.

In addition to Aseptoplast lenses' biostatic properties against gram-positive bacteria, the lenses were more wettable. This led to efforts to increase wettability in other modified polymer plastics resulting in WJ Type "A." Type "A" exhibited increased wettability properties compared to the standard materials.

To help patients identify the right contact lens from the left contact lens, Wesley-Jessen offered the Lumicon® lens identification mark, which was a small dark blue or black dot placed on the edge of either the right or left lens, whichever was preferred. Of course, this is unnecessary if the two eye powers were identical or if the fit was the same. If the powers were different slightly or the fitting properties between the two lenses different, then the Lumicon dot was helpful for patients. Dots were applied for other positional purposes such as cylinder location or prism ballast positions.

Contact Lens Curiosities

Newton Wesley was always fascinated by anything related to eyes. He collected many items related to vision and eyes, which he placed in his museum.

Dr. Wesley and his staff created ruby-red contact lenses to identify marked playing cards. The original thought behind the ruby-red color was that they might help those afflicted by red-green color-blindness to enhance their perception of color. There was a limited enhancement, so they abandoned the project. The ruby-red contacts went on to be a novelty product.

The National Eye Research Foundation held annual meetings

in Las Vegas, Nevada. Some company employees thought it would be fun to develop contact lenses to beat the system. They made the lenses and cards in jest, but some people took it seriously and tried to build and promote the concept. The ruby-red contact lenses could identify marked playing cards that invisibly identified the cards' suit and value on the back of the card. The giveaway that made it impossible to use in the real world was the fact that the person trying to cheat wore red contact lenses. They could be easily identified just by looking at their eyes. The tricky concept has not gone away. Today, invisible ink-marked cards are available, along with regular contact lenses that make the marking visible.

Bifocal Contact Lens Designs

Ideas for contact lens designs came from many sources in Newton's world of vision. In Newton Wesley's private collection were two eyeglasses with slits. One pair was made of Polynesian wood and another of white plastic. Both pairs of glasses have thin rectangular slits at the level of the pupil. These curious "glasses" derive from concepts whose origin is lost in time. In extremely bright areas of the planet, people have sought protection for their eyes and an ability to improve their vision under these conditions. Eskimos needed to protect their eyes from the bright glaring snow and to evaluate better snow conditions where subtle differences can mean disaster or survival. Habitants in sunny environments such as the desert need protection from those harsh conditions. Eyeglasses with slits were the answer in both situations.

Eyeglasses with slits were probably invented sometime after the pinhole effect was noticed, which helped provide better vision. A pin can be used to make a small hole in a sheet of dark paper. The pinhole is held up in front of one eye with the other closed. Vision is improved because the incoming rays of light to the eye are restricted. The small hole eliminates extraneous light rays that blur vision. Also, Newton's collection had a variety of "lenses" with pinholes to improve visual acuity.

The principle of restricting the light rays coming into the central portion of the eye was applied to contact lens design. Newton had many types of lenses made that attempted to improve vision using various patterns on the lens. Here are some of the lenses designed that were made in an attempt to find the best design that would improve vision. These designs were applications of the pinhole principle.

Benjamin Franklin was the inventor of bifocal glasses to allow people to read who had a visual problem called presbyopia ("old age" sight). Attempts to make contact lenses with the same Franklin design bifocal were an early method to correct near-reading

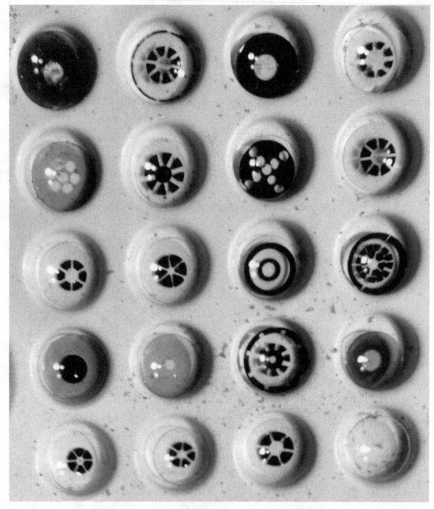

Wesley-Jessen designs for bifocal and multifocal lenses.

problems with contact lenses. Fused bifocal contact lenses were made by the ophthalmologist Chester Black and WJ's lab manager Joseph Cinefro in the 1950s. These bifocal contact lenses could help those with near-reading problems.

Multifocal contact lenses were later designed with a continuously changing curvature to increase the reading power as the contact moved down the eye into reading positions.

10 NERF AND THE FIRST INTERNATIONAL CONTACT LENS CONGRESS

By 1959, NERF's membership grew large enough to hold the First Contact Lens Congress at the Edgewater Beach Hotel in Chicago. Over 2,000 people attended the three day August meeting near the shores of Lake Michigan, attracting speakers and registrants from around the world. A 65 page Press Book was distributed in advance to national newspapers, magazines, radio, and television stations. The NERF Press Book provided ready to use media information on meeting research topics, contact lens survey information, and human interest stories with photographs.

Some data that was presented in the NERF Press Book:

Industry Growth 1950 to 1959

	Wearers	Practitioners	Laboratories
1950	200,000	1,000	Less than 20
1957	3,000,000	9,000	35
1958	4,075,946	12,000	More than 35
1959	6,660,096*	15,600	112

*64.7% are females, or 4.33 million / 35.3% are males, or 2.33 million

Increase in contact lens services by contact lens fitters

	% Contact Lens	% Other Eye Care Services
1957	5	95
1958	22	78
1959	50	50

Adaptation Time: General opinion is that it takes three and a half weeks to adjust to contact lenses. They could then be worn with the same "taken for grantedness" as an article of clothing, belt, earring, etc.

Adult Reasons for Wearing Contact Lenses

Women	Men
Vanity (79.3%)	Masculine Ego (39.4%)
Social Acceptance	Convenience
Better Vision	Better Vision
Male Influence	Athletic Activities
Convenience	Occupational Reasons
Athletic Activities	Social Acceptance
"Vogue"	"Newest Thing"

Separate press releases were sent out to focus attention on special interest features such as the fashion dresses made with thousands of contact lenses embroidered into the fabric worn by the German model and actress, Anne-Marie Kolb. Worldwide news stories featured her wearing the contact lens dress that was insured for a million dollars by Lloyd's of London.

Columnist Robert Herguth wrote an article in the July 29, 1959, *Chicago Daily News,* titled "$1 Million Dress Is Something to See" stating,

> Carrying a million dollar dress and $25 worth of underwear, beautiful Anne-Marie Kolb got off the plane at Midway Airport Wednesday. "The dress is made of 10,000 contact lenses," explained Ann-Marie, a German actress who is quite a spectacle herself. "I wore another dress on the flight from New York because did you ever try to sit down in a dress made of contact lenses?" Everybody shook their heads, "no." What do you wear underneath a plastic dress worth $1 million, Anne-Marie was asked. "Not too much." She explained that not much underwear cost $25 because it came from Paris.
>
> Q. What does such a dress feel like to wear?
>
> A. Gemütlich. Cozy.
>
> Q. How do you clean a dress made of 10,000 contact lenses?
>
> A. It hasn't got dirty yet. I guess I will have to buy some window cleaner. It's windy.

Q. The dress is windy?

A. No, Chicago is windy. Do you think I will be able to see Chicago 5,000 times as well in a dress of 10,00 plastic lenses?

Ann Marie, who wears plastic lenses over her blue eyes, is in town to be crowned Miss International Contact Lens Monday at the First World Contact Lens Congress in the Edgewater Beach hotel.

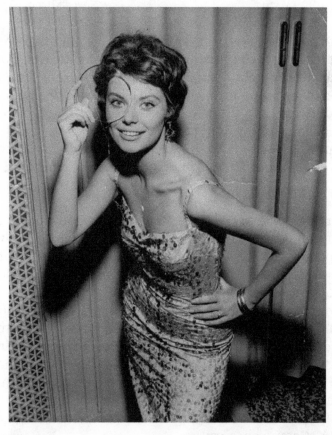

Miss International Contact Lens, Anne-Marie Kolb of Germany wearing the "Million Dollar Contact Lens Dress" insured by Lloyds of London, November 1959. (Press release photo, Roy Wesley personal collection)

The million dollar dress was designed and made by dressmaker Gladyce (Gladys) Filer of Chicago. She also created and made six outfits to be worn at various Congress events, including men's ties and cuff links with a distinctive script design "Contact Lenses."

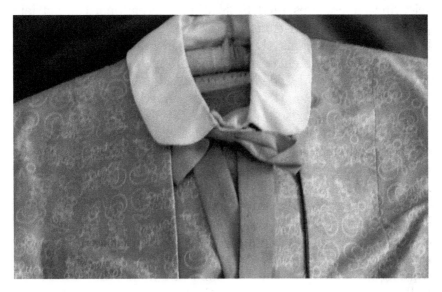

Gladys Filer Script Contact Lenses designer dress for day wear, 1959. (Roy Wesley personal collection)

Contacto described the opening day:

> A flag ceremony on Sunday, August 2, will mark the official opening of the Congress, with the presence of civic officials, a dedication reading, and salute to the flags of the United States, United Nations, Eye Research Foundation, and the City of Chicago. On Sunday night, the first evening of the Congress, a cocktail and dinner party in Old Western-style will show visitors from other countries the American side of fun, food, and music. A special presentation will be made of an American institution ... the hot dog ... and for some, it will be the first-ever eaten. During the second Congress night, a banquet, with after-dinner dancing, will feature an

all-nation atmosphere. Civic officials and celebrities will share the dais during an entertainment packed program. ("Edgewater Beach meeting," 1959, p. 131)

The daytime program of the International Congress featured 30 scientific papers presented by leading international contact lens practitioners. An IBM translator system, similar to the one used by the United Nations (UN), offered instantaneous translation from speaker to listener. Closed-circuit television allowed close observation of technical demonstrations without interference.

It was the first time UN interpreters served outside their regular assignments. It was also the first time German and Japanese were added to Russian, French, and Spanish, which made up the official UN languages with English and Chinese. The United Nations was founded in 1945 in San Francisco and located in New York City in 1948.

Istvan Gyorffy, MD, from Budapest, spoke on "Contact lens fitting in Hungary," and was the keynote presenter. Gyorffy worked at Josef Dallos' London clinic and was an early developer using PMMA to make scleral lenses (1937). In his lecture, he described working in isolation in Hungary following the methods of Joseph Dallos for fitting contact lenses. He said, "My modification was to use acrylate instead of glass as the material for the shells. ...I succeeded in finding a pressing process and grinding method for accurate lens production and, in the early months of 1939, I was able to supply a small part of my patients with contact lenses."

Other international presenters were:

Peter Ruseski, MD, who gave results of a year long contact lens study in the Antarctic illustrating contact lens experiments under extreme conditions at the Byrd Station and elsewhere.

Jan Vanýsek, MD, from Czechoslovakia, reported on contacts used for diagnostic and cosmetic purposes. He established the first contact lens laboratory and ophthalmology clinic in Hradec Kralove, Czechoslovakia and was a pioneer of intraocular implants.

Mme. R Koch, Paris, France, ophthalmology student of early contact lens pioneer R.A. Dudragne, spoke on the use of contact lenses in keratoconus.

Professor Tutomu Sato, MD from Juntendo University, Tokyo, presented his case histories on 30 young patients 8 months to 10 years old illustrating correction or retardation of strabismus by contact lens applications.

Hernando Henao of Bogota, Columbia, discussed the application of contact lenses after corneal transplants to correct irregular vision following surgery.

There were relevant programs for the doctors, their assistants, staff, as well as doctors' wives and families. The meeting tried to include everyone associated with an eye care practice.

NERF educational meetings reached a peak of influence from 1960-1970 when Congresses were held in Las Vegas, Nevada, where Hollywood stars were featured. NERF tapped into the trend and began to have stars like the comedian, Bob Newhart at the November, 1970 National meeting. Sammy Davis, Junior appeared at the 16th National Eye Research Congress at the Sands Hotel. Much of the inspiration for using these stars as features for the meeting came from that chance encounter Newton had in meeting Phyllis Diller in Chicago at the Palmer House in the 1950s.

The growth of contact lenses and increased revenues to the eye doctors' practices allowed them to indulge themselves and their families in new adventures. Eye care professionals profited from this new addition to their sales, as did Wesley-Jessen and other manufacturers of contacts.

Evenings were highlighted by banquets and award ceremonies. José Ferrer, Hollywood actor, broadway star, and director, was the master of ceremonies for the World Contact Lens Congress Banquet. *Contacto* (1959) wrote that "speaking fluently in seven languages, he will be able to greet delegates in their native tongue." José Ferrer had won an Oscar in 1950 for his role in the film "Cyrano de Bergerac" and had won several Tony awards. At the time of the event, Mr. Ferrer's wife was the singer and actress Rosemary Clooney. The use of Hollywood stars as a draw for the national meetings was in keeping with the times and the increased affluence and interests of optometrists.

Miss America beauty contests began in 1921. In the 1950s, the beauty competition was an American institution popularized by television. NERF borrowed the glamour and allure of the beauty contest at its meeting. The image and symbolism of Miss America has changed significantly over 100 years. At the time of the Congress, there was a strong appeal of the idealized female to the mostly male audience of optometrists. In addition to the jury selection of German actress Anne-Marie Kolb as Miss International Contact Lens, another beauty, Miss Anne Robinson, was chosen from the United States as Miss USA Contact Lens. Anne Robinson was Miss Virginia in the Miss America beauty pageant.

Comments of support for the First World Congress were received from Presidents Dwight D. Eisenhower and Richard Nixon and were used at the opening of the meeting:

"I extend greetings to the participants of the 1st World Contact Lens Congress in Chicago, Illinois. You have my best in your chosen specialty." *-Dwight D. Eisenhower*

"I welcome this opportunity to send my best wishes to all of the representatives from 34 nations in attendance for a most stimulating and effective conference and for continued success in their efforts to achieve better vision for all people." *-Richard Nixon*

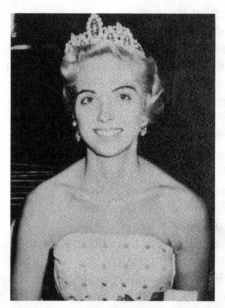

Miss USA Contact Lens, Anne Robinson

It was a culmination of years of training, inventions, and development of techniques and ideas in fitting lenses, advertising, and marketing to doctors and the public. The Edgewater Beach Hotel in 1959 still had a nostalgic charm to the attendees of the meeting. Chicago's Lake Michigan's waves came to the back of the small sandy beach at the back of the hotel up until 1951 when Lake Shore Drive was extended and expanded to the north and east, cutting off access to the lake. The sprawling pink hotel complex was reminiscent of a Florida beach resort with the ocean replaced by Lake Michigan. Hollywood entertainers such as Charlie Chaplin, Judy Garland, and Frank Sinatra played there or were guests, and big bands like Benny Goodman, Tommy Dorsey, and Glenn Miller were featured. The Edgewater Beach was also conveniently located just a few blocks from Newton Wesley's home, a new development glass apartment building to the north.

This First World Contact Lens Congress was such a success that Newton and the company began to plan immediately for the next big event three years later. The next World Congress was announced one month afterward in the September 1959 issue of *Contacto*. By November 1959, the special edition of *Contacto* announced "Vision '62" as the next event, the First World Vision Exposition in Chicago. The staff selected the newly constructed McCormick Place Exposition Center in Chicago as the venue. The Foundation team planned and executed three different regional meetings during the same year of the World Congress. Local congresses were to be held in New York City at the Roosevelt Hotel on November 2-3, 1959, in Chicago on November 9-10 at the Sherman Hotel, and on November 16-17 in San Francisco's Sheraton Palace Hotel. These were large undertakings for the relatively small staff of NERF employees then operating out of the 11th-floor offices at the Champlain Building, 37 South Wabash Avenue in Chicago. At the time, the manufacturing laboratories of Wesley-Jessen expanded to two floors, the 8th and 9th, of the same building. This pace of meetings was unsustainable and costly, so eventually, the decision was made to consolidate meetings and present one annual National Meeting in Las Vegas, Nevada. NERF held meetings in Las Vegas for 25 years after that.

Newton's partner in business, George N. Jessen, made the decision to retire from Wesley-Jessen and the clinic practice he led at Jessen-Wesley in 1969 after the tragic loss of his first grandchild.

However, he explained his retirement to those at the company in his characteristic style:

> *With all of the papers in this envelope, you have one that says in sort of cold legal language that Doctor Jessen intends to go into partial retirement.*
>
> *I guess that I can say without any fear of contradiction, as the years have gone by, we have all aged a day or so. Even my buddy, Newton, has said that he has to slow up a little bit, but from the schedule that he keeps, I don't see that he has. For my part, these doggone Chicago winters seem to have been getting longer and colder and tougher to live with, and since I have been in them for a fairly sufficient number of years, I somehow felt that it wasn't necessary to continue to fight them. As a matter of fact, Lillian and I have purchased a home in the sunny State of Nevada, and while the rest of you younger "fellas" are struggling with the snow and ice here in Chicago, I hope to be at least working in the sunshine of Nevada.* (Jessen, 1969)

He was 53 years old and moved with his wife, Lillian, to a home at the edge of a Las Vegas golf course. He lived another 18 years but succumbed to liver cancer due to a hepatitis C infection obtained on a trip to China before a vaccine was available. Because of the annual NERF meetings in Las Vegas, Newton was able to stay in touch with George and Lillian for many years after his retirement. Even though George and Newton never had a legal written agreement to their partnership, Newton always felt they were partners. At the time of the sale in 1980, Newton gave half of the proceeds to George in recognition of their partnership.

Contacto and WJ Publications

Wesley-Jessen published many instructional and educational pamphlets for eye doctors and patients. Newton met Martin Topaz, the publisher at the Professional Press located across the street from WJ at 5 North Wabash in the historic 1910 Kesner building where another famous publisher, Arch W. Shaw had his headquarters. Martin followed in his father Lionel Topaz' publishing footsteps. Lionel published the *Optometric Weekly* (1910), *The Optician,* and books in ophthalmology and optometry. The Topaz family and WJ were aided by the fact that Chicago was a printing hub in the United States with many printers located one mile south in Printer's Row. Wesley-Jessen published *Contacto* beginning in 1957 with Leonard Bronstein, OD, as editor and an editorial board consisting of Neal J. Bailey, OD from Indiana University's Optometry School; Chester Black, MD; Frederick E. Farnum, OD from Boston; and Robert W. Lester, OD, from San Francisco. *Contacto* was the first journal of contact lenses published in the United States (Goss, 2018, p. 52).

Neal J. Bailey, OD, PhD (1917-2006) was a contemporary of Newton Wesley with a similar background for entering optometry and the eye care field in that both had eye problems that distorted their vision significantly and needed solutions. Neal Bailey had severe astigmatism, and Newton Wesley had keratoconus. Neal Bailey was a professor at Ohio State University and had an optometric practice on campus, which specialized in contact lenses beginning in 1958. Half of his practice were patients with keratoconus or aphakia (the condition of the eye after the internal lens is removed during cataract surgery). He became an associate editor of *Contacto.* Later he became the first editor of *Contact Lens Forum,* and he initiated the journal *Contact Lens Spectrum,* which absorbed Contact Lens Forum in time. In 1987, Bailey published the 100th Anniversary edition of *Contact Lens Spectrum* devoted to the history of contact lenses using the Wiesbaden 1887 molded glass lens that Newton obtained and purchased in Germany in 1956. This lens became the prototype of the earliest contact lens. In a chronicle of historical development, Bailey had a chapter on "Wesley and Jessen: Industry Pioneers." He began the article with a personal story that demonstrated the teaching commitment that Newton had and his dedication to training eye doctors.

The year was 1945, the place Chicago. Standing before Newton K. Wesley, OD, cursing like a cowboy, was the first of some 25,000 'students' to follow over the years. Having observed, questioned, and pestered Dr. Wesley for a week about his contact lens work, the East Texas OD wanted to know how much he owed Wesley for his time and instructions. 'Nothing,' answered Wesley. Up until then,

Wesley hadn't considered the broader implications of his and his partner's single-minded research in contact lenses. 'You don't realize that what you've taught me is worth thousands of dollars!' Wesley remembers his first student barking. The earlier curse words weren't meant to defame, but to serve as a pat on the back. Dr. Wesley and his partner, George N. Jessen, OD, progressed from giving practical advice to brain-pickers to pioneering the development and introduction of contact lenses worldwide. For at least the first quarter-century of the modern contact lens era, the two were virtually synonymous with the term contact lenses.

This comment is high praise from one well-acquainted with the contact lens industry from the inside. Bailey continued describing the origins of the NERF journal *Contacto*:

In January 1957, the Eye Research Foundation put together a group which, in turn, put together the materials for the January 1957, Vol. 1, No. 1, issue of *Contacto*, its "official house publication." I was on the first board of editorial advisors. Many of the Eye Research Foundation congresses held in Chicago convened at the Edgewater Beach Hotel, a plush "in" place of the 1950s. Each of the first four annual meetings was more exciting and larger than the previous one, and 1959 was the 'peak' meeting with over 1,000 in attendance. Constantly new ideas, new designs, new promotions, and new faces kept these meetings vitally in tune with contact lens progress. In June 1960, the Eye Research Foundation became the National Eye Research Foundation (NERF) and is known by this latter name today.

Bailey concluded with a description of the "downfall" of NERF:

By 1960, however, a great deal of the earlier "newness" - engendered enthusiasm began to wane, and the NERF meetings and the NERF organization itself began to falter, partly because of the disfavor into which it fell, especially with the schools. It was looked upon purely as the public relations arm of the Plastic Contact Lens Company. Unfortunate as the above facts may be, the Wesley-Jessen team deserves high praise. Two men (plus the "team" or "teams" they assembled nationally and internationally) found themselves at a time in history that needed their talents. They proceeded to propel the contact lens from a little-known—but perhaps much-sought-after—device fitted by a minority of eye care practitioners to an amazingly well-known vision device fitted by a majority of eye care practitioners. Carried to the public on radio programs, TV programs, newspapers, and magazines, the National Eye Research Foundation, the names Newton Wesley and George Jessen, and the contact lens products they mentioned became household words. The field of contact lenses benefitted and continues even today to benefit from the promotional efforts of this pair of entrepreneurs. (Bailey, 1987, pp. 2-64)

Neal Bailey's comments of NERF's decline starting in 1960 may be premature. It seems the following decade began the descent with the introduction of the soft lens. Wesley-Jessen and NERF were clearly on the rise in the 1960s. Still, they had spawned steady competition from manufacturers entering the field, optometry schools offering competing continuing education credits, and professional organizations providing contact lens courses at their meetings. It was inevitable that the large market share that WJ and NERF had was to decline over time.

On the lighter side, one of Wesley-Jessen's publications to reach the public was a book of 28 contact lens cartoons called *Sphertoons*, published in 1957. Each cartoon came with a factoid about contact lenses for public information under the cartoon caption. The cartoons were illustrated by artist Bob Markowitz from ideas generated by Newton, George and long time associate Bette Bagnel. The opening of the booklet stated, "Today with over 2,000,000 Americans wearing Contact Lenses ... the humorists are having a field day ... as illustrated by the cartoons assembled for your amusement." The centerfold of the cartoon book listed prominent people wearing contact lenses. Among them were Ronald Reagan, Ester Williams, Deborah Kerr, Bill McColl (Chicago Bears), Frank Gifford (NY Giants), and Kyle Rote (NY Giants).

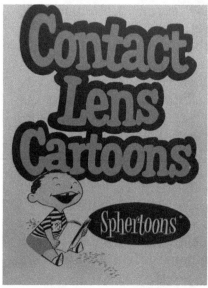 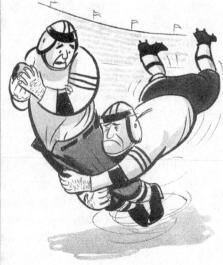

"*Put your contact lenses on, Spike; I'm on your team.*"

LEFT: Cover of Sphertoons, Contact Lens Cartoons (1957); RIGHT: One of the 26 cartoons. (Roy Wesley personal collection)

International Wesley-Jessen

About 1956, Newton received an invitation from well known Professor Tsutomo Sato of the Tokyo Juntendo University department of ophthalmology to lecture on contact lenses. Professor Sato was a student of Shinobu Ishihara, the doctor famous for developing the Ishihara Color Vision Test, which became a worldwide standard. Not only was Sato a student of Ishihara, but he was also related to him because he married his daughter. Sato was also the personal eye doctor to the Emperor of Japan and his family. Dr. Sato had an interest in contact lenses in 1934 when he made some glass scleral lenses. He abandoned the effort when the superior Carl Zeiss lenses were sold in Japan. Shortly after Newton declined Professor Sato's invitation, he received a phone call from a St. Louis ophthalmologist, Dr. Tsuyoshi Yamashita, who inquired why Newton refused Professor Sato's invitation. Dr. Yamashita was a colleague and student of Dr. Sato and was asked to intercede on his behalf to get Newton to come to Japan. Newton realized that he was being rude to the respected Dr. Sato and continued discussions with Dr. Yamashita to determine if Newton could give a lecture in Japanese. Newton learned to speak Japanese from his immigrant parents, but it was the language spoken half a century ago. Dr. Sato arranged for a crash course in Japanese in Hakone where Newton could concentrate on perfecting his language skills with a medical student that Dr. Sato provided. Newton wrote:

> Professor Sato and I got along very well. He had mapped out an itinerary for me. He wanted me to study in his favorite mountain retreat near Hakone at the base of Mount Fuji. He assured me that I would have privacy and that he would assign a medical student to me, a Dr. Komatsu. I could get by conversationally, but my problem was how I was going to say: "Cataract or dystrophy or retinitis pigments?" The technical language threw me completely. He said he understood. He felt my studies should be completed within the three weeks before the meetings and that I would have to study very hard. I told him I was very grateful and that I would do my best. He set up a morning for me to see patients at the hospital. He wanted me to examine them and fit them with my contact lenses–the Sphercon, to which I agreed and the date was set. (Wesley, 1988, p. 141)

Since this was Newton Wesley's first trip to Japan, Dr. Sato provided tours in Hakone and Tokyo as well as tickets to traditional Noh drama, so that he could be introduced to the culture his parents left.

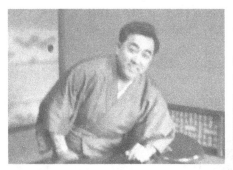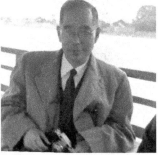

Dr. Newton K. Wesley (left) and Dr. Tsutomu Sato (right), 1957 meeting in Hakone, Japan. (Roy Wesley personal collection)

Newton attended tea ceremonies and Zen gardens to absorb Japanese tranquility and harmony. He was a perplexed tourist on the Tokyo bus tour named "Pigeon Bus Company," surrounded by symbols of peace until he realized that it was a subtle mistranslation of the Japanese word hato, which could be a pigeon or dove. They chose the wrong bird to represent peace in English. He could be tolerant because he would make similar mistakes in trying to convey English words rendered into Japanese during his lecture which would provoke gentle laughter.

His lecture was delivered successfully in the town of Gifu, famous for its cormorant fishing birds. The 1957 Japanese Ophthalmological Society meeting brought in 5,000 doctors for his 15-minute lecture in Japanese. Later in the day, Newton spoke for 2 hours to a small group of 200 medical researchers. Dr. Shinichi Shimizu was president and organizer of the Society's 61st meeting and was also the Gifu University Ophthalmology Department's Chairman. Dr. Sato arranged for Newton to visit the historic cities of Kyoto and Nara following the meetings accompanied by Dr. Hikaru Hamano as his guide. Following the tour, Newton gave a Sphercon fitting course to a group of 40 highly respected ophthalmologists for several days. The presentation included fourteen patients that Dr. Sato requested Newton fit with his trial Sphercon lenses the previous month upon his arrival in Tokyo. Newton reported,

> The professors began to question them and check them with their equipment, including the slit lamp.... I was amazed to learn that even under the very difficult circumstances that I had fitted the patients on my second day in Japan at Juntendo University, all were wearing their lenses all day long.... The professors were amazed and happy that all fourteen cases were successful (Wesley, 1988, p. 149)

Professor Sato told Newton that he could hardly understand one word of his Japanese at the beginning of his visit, but that after the last week of lectures and patient visits, he understood every word. Professor Sato introduced Newton to the president of Juntendo University and found that part of the reason he was invited to Japan was that the president's daughter wanted to wear contact lenses but could not be fitted by the Japanese fitters. Newton proved to them that contact lenses could be properly fitted. Sato also introduced Newton to his famous father-in-law, Professor Ishikawa. Dr. Sato had related to Ishikawa Newton's generosity in coming to Japan for a month at his own expense, giving lectures, and fitting patients. Ishikawa responded by presenting to Newton a simple Japanese kanji character, *jin*, 人類, expressing the concept "for the good of humanity." Newton said,

> It was his way of saying thank you to me, because I had given of myself. I had donated my lecture fees, my travel costs to the Japanese, because I thought they needed them more than I did. I even gave them the rights to the Sphercon patent in Japan. Professor Sato and the manufacturer there combined forces. Interestingly, the coalition was so strong that I couldn't get back into Japan as a manufacturer. In fact, I really didn't try. (Wesley, 1988, p. 151)

Newton continued teaching contact lens fitting practices and manufacturing procedures to the Japanese after this opening. In 1967, for example, he made a trip to Asia to deliver training courses in Japan to the Japan Contact Lens Research Society and in the Philippines (see photos in Appendix). In recognition of Dr. Wesley's lectures and Sphercon training sessions from 1973, he received a gold medal from the Japanese Ophthalmological Society.

Through his work in Japan, Newton developed a strong bond and personal relationship with Hikaru Hamano, MD, of Osaka, Japan. As an ophthalmologist, Dr. Hamano attended the 1957 lecture that Newton gave in Japan and felt the need to devote his practice to contact lenses as a specialty practice. He was the first Japanese ophthalmologist to devote his practice to contact lenses. In so doing, he established one of the largest and most successful contact lens clinics in Japan. He not only saw patients but was always interested in the medical aspects of contact lens fittings and has published many articles and books on corneal physiology and contact lenses. Hikaru Hamano would sometimes fly from Japan to Chicago to attend special family events for Newton, and Newton would visit Hikaru at his home in Osaka. This close relationship allowed Newton to obtain his Doctor of Medicine degree from Osaka University, a research degree awarded based on his work in developing Photo Electric Keratoscopy (PEK), a method of mapping the cornea to aid in the fitting of contact lenses. This work was carried out at Wesley-Jessen and resulted in the manufacture and sales of the PEK instrument that doctors used in their practice to map the cornea to help improve contact lens fits. In particular, PEK was used to determine the topographical shape of the cornea before a contact lens was fitted. PEK illustrated the topography of the cornea so the contact lens could be accurately matched. This comparative analysis could lead to improved fitting and better comfort for the patient.

Newton's family visited Dr. Hamano and his family in Osaka in 1970, at which time Dr. Hamano arranged for a VIP tour of the Osaka 1970 World Exposition. Dr. Hamano provided a one month tour of Japan for Dr. Wesley's two sons. They were accompanied by two of Hamano's clinic assistants, Miss Ayako and Miss Hamamoto, who served as guides and translators. This trip was a generosity that reflected Dr. Hamano's gratitude for Dr. Wesley's guidance and friendship in establishing Hamano's Osaka eye clinic. Dr. Hamano flew to Portland for Newton's mother's funeral in 1962 and assisted him with his father's funeral arrangements in Gobo City, Wakayama, Japan in 1966. Newton visited Dr. Hamano and his family many times in Japan after their meeting in 1957. Through the last 54 years of Newton's life, they were close friends, colleagues, and supporters of each other's endeavors.

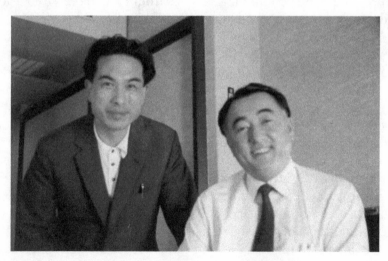

Dr. Hikaru Hamano and Dr. Newton Wesley, Osaka, Japan, 1968. (Roy Wesley personal collection)

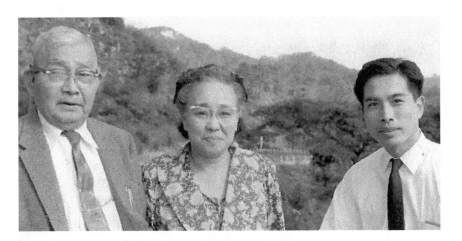

Newton's parents Kojiro and Chiyo Uyesugi with Dr. Hamano, Wakayama, Japan. (Roy Wesley personal collection)

11 ORTHOKERATOLOGY AND MYOPIA CONTROL

The term "orthokeratology" was created by Dr. Wesley at a NERF meeting in Chicago, as described by Joseph Nolan at the first meeting of the International Orthokeratology Society (IOS). George Jessen preferred to use the term "orthofocus" to mean the same thing, but orthokeratology is the term in current use. Orthokeratology (Ortho-K, OK) and myopia control may be defined as the correction and improvement of vision using contact lenses. Orthokeratology does not use surgical intervention. *Ortho* is the Greek prefix meaning correct, straight, or upright. Keratology, as used in this context, means the study of the cornea. *Keras* is the Greek word for horn. Since animal horns are made of protein, modern usage refers to proteins such as the transparent collagen layer in the eye's cornea. Thus, orthokeratology's original meaning was intended to be the "correct shaping of the cornea" using contact lenses.

Many men have been listed as "the father of orthokeratology." H.A. Swarbrick (2006) stated, "The father of modern orthokeratology is undoubtedly George Jessen" (p. 125). Dr. Wesley is considered by some to be the originator of orthokeratogy. However, Dr. George Jessen is most often cited as "the father of orthokeratology" in the literature. Numerous men were working together in the first think tank of orthokeratology: Joseph Nolan, Charles May, Stuart Grant, Donald Harris, Al Fontana, Richard Wlodyga, Nick Stoyan, Sami El Hage, John Reinhart, Roger Tabb, John Mountford, Cary Herzberg, and many others. Given Dr. Joseph Nolan's 1962 credit to Dr. Wesley coining the word orthokeratology, it would seem that Dr. Newton Wesley should be among those considered for the title of "Father of Orthokeratology."

Since the earliest days of fitting the microlens developed by Wilhelm Söhnges and the microlens created by Wesley-Jessen, a central flattening of the cornea due to the fitting techniques of the time resulted in an unintentional orthokeratology or vision improvement when the contact lens was removed. The contact lens' base curve was fitted flatter than the central curvature of the patient's cornea. The resultant corneal flattening sometimes resulted in improved vision in myopes (nearsighted people) that lasted from minutes to hours after lens removal. This feature has been developed over the years, with orthokeratology being developed simultaneously with new plastic polymers, lens geometry modifications, improved fitting techniques, and scientific research resulting in better, longer-lasting visual improvement.

Newton fostered the spirit of research in orthokeratology and was instrumental in establishing a section of the National Eye Research Foundation devoted to the subject. The first meeting of the International Orthokeratology Section (IOS) was held in 1962 in conjunction with a NERF meeting in Chicago. This organization led to the growth of the field, spawned many other organizations globally, and has led to significant research in myopia control. IOS members published their work in various optometric journals. They compiled their work and new research in 1972 when the journal *Orthokeratology* was launched under the leadership of Stuart Grant, Charles May, and Joseph Nolan. A paper on myopia control was first published in *Orthokeratology* in 1976 in an article "Myopia Control Now" by Donald Harris. Dr. Harris' interest in myopia control began when he worked in Point Barrow, Alaska in 1968. He noted that "Only two eyes were found to be nearsighted in an adult Eskimo population of 130. But after an educational system was instituted for the Eskimos, 60% of the children of those 130 adults were myopic." The underlying causes of myopia development and its prevention in children became a concern for many orthokeratologists in IOS.

Orthokeratology (OK) is part of the myopia control movement in eye care. Recent research has moved the field from the cornea's haphazard flattening to measuring and understanding corneal shape during the process. Doctors now take computer-generated topographic maps of the cornea before and after fitting OK lenses. Observing the contours of three-dimensional mapping permits greater control of the fit and final result of 20/20 vision without glasses or contacts. New oxygen permeable plastic contact lenses allow for more extended wear during the day and even for lenses worn overnight. Computer-designed OK lenses with multiple aspheric curves control the corneal shape and provide longer-lasting vision than previously obtained.

Dr. Newton Wesley would appreciate the new developments applied to his keratoconus using the new computer-assisted fitting techniques, gas permeable lenses designed by computers, and manufactured by computer-controlled lathes. His early research using computers to generate corneal maps (PEK) and contact lenses helped to lead the way to the developments that exist in the industry today.

12 EPILOGUE

Newton Wesley learned skills from his childhood experiences that prepared him uniquely for facing and controlling future business adversities. Playing, hunting, and fishing with his many cousins and friends in Westport's forests taught him to cooperate with others to achieve common goals. Hard work raising plants on his father's Sherwood farm provided insights into crop success and failure. Newton applied all these experiences in business management as he developed his company. His urbanized education in Portland provided the tools to explore and survive in cities and corporate life. From his early judo experiences, Newton embodied the Japanese concept of Satoyama 里山 and Judo 柔道 (the gentle way). In facing challenging situations in life, he applied the philosophy of not resisting and going with the flow to achieve a desired outcome. He learned a lesson of strength and achievement as a young boy swimming with the river flow to an island in the middle of the Columbia River off the shores of the lumber mill camp where he grew up.

Newton did not spend as much time as a family man compared with the average man of his generation—the "Leave It To Beaver" type of dad. He was not the dad to come home from work and always be there with the family at breakfast, dinner, and weekends. He was a "family businessman" who often said, "The reason I work so hard is for my family." At the same time, he incorporated his business life into his family.

The business was part of his family. Employees and clients became intimates woven into the fabric of his family life. It was common to have dinners and events with doctors who were Wesley-Jessen clients or with workers from the company mixed in with family members.

The annual company picnic and other outings were a fun way to bring workers and their families together on a Sunday afternoon outing. Saturday was still a lab production workday for some, so Sunday was a time when all workers, their families, and friends could take off in the afternoon. Chicago's Northwest side Forest Preserve LaBagh Woods at Cicero and Foster was a convenient site for company picnics. Workers volunteered to bring picnic foods and organize baseball and other games for everyone of all ages.

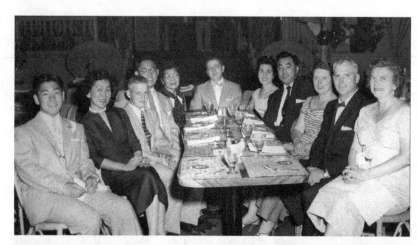

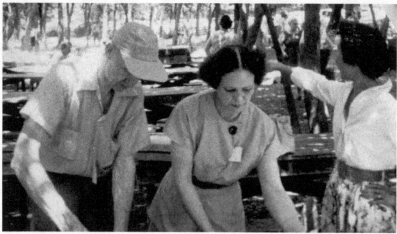

TOP: Family and Wesley-Jessen dinner at the Edgewater Beach Hotel Polynesian Room, 1956. Roy Wesley, Cecilia Wesley, Michael Jessen, Lee Wesley, Yae Sasaki, Edmund Janies, Jan Janies, Newton K. Wesley, Lillian Jessen, George Jessen, Majorie Fournier. BOTTOM: Wesley-Jessen Annual picnic, LaBagh Woods picnic grove, North Park Chicago, Ca 1955. Mr. and Mrs. Ray Urban, Mrs. Cecilia Wesley (Roy Wesley personal collection).

Newton folded his real family into his business life in many ways. During the early 1950s, Newton traveled to visit doctors to train and gain sales. Some of these trips became family outings, with packed lunches for the drive, and meals with doctors or clients. Sometimes business meetings were held at home or well-known restaurants downtown. On rare occasions, Newton brought his family on vacations to distant shores like Europe or the Orient while he did business.

The sense of family in business became a corporate legacy passed on from his leadership to future generations of WJ presidents. They continued to have company outings, picnics, and parties to give employees a sense of belonging to a company that cared about them and their participation in common goals. A WJ Reunion held in Arlington Heights, IL, July 2018, with 300 former employees, celebrated the spirit of belonging and experiencing the joy of working in a unique company environment. Jim Moritz was the prime organizer of the reunion.

Newton influenced his family members to become optometrists, even his wife, Cecilia, who attended Monroe College of Optometry when Newton taught there. Newton inspired his younger brother, Edward Uyesugi, to pursue optometry as a career after Ed graduated from Earlham College. Edward graduated from Northern Illinois College of Optometry (NICO) in 1949. He created a unique and controversial low vision practice in Paoli, Indiana, that helped many struggling to preserve or enhance their vision using contact lenses. The controversial part of his method was his application of high plus contact lenses on low vision patients. He tried to create an accommodative push to force the eye to work harder to see through the blur. Dr. Uyesugi's clinic sign in Paoli read,

Dr. E.T. UYESUGI, Inc. OPTOMETRIC CLINIC.
Specializing in Contact Lenses, Orthokeratology, Low
Vision, Preventive Eye Care

Newton and Edward's sister Corinne married Terrence Toda. Terrence (Terry) became an optometrist after graduating from Southern College of Optometry (Memphis, TN) and practiced in Seattle, WA. Corinne and Terry had two daughters, Jerilyn and Alyce. Jerilyn Toda attended Pacific College of Optometry to become a practicing doctor. She married an optometrist, Lund Chin. They practiced at Terrence Toda's Seattle Vision Clinic. Jerilyn and Lund had two sons, Brent and Gregory, who became optometrists upon graduation from the Pacific College of Optometry. In Newton's immediate family, his son Roy Wesley received his OD from New England College of Optometry. Newton's daughter, Jenna Wesley (offspring of his second marriage), graduated from Illinois College of Optometry. Newton's older son, Lee Wesley, was President of the WJ Spectacle Division in Champaign, Illinois, and worked in the Research Department developing soft lens products.

Newton's first wife, Cecilia, passed away on August 22, 1973, at 56, suffering five years from stomach cancer's ravages. It was difficult for Newton to lose his wife of 33 years after starting life with her following the Great Depression, through the war years, and re-starting life in Chicago. The funeral service and interment were held two days following her death. Newton flew to Boston to lead a seminar on PEK for doctors on the next day. Newton's characteristic was to do the work he saw necessary at the moment during various life crises. When Japan attacked America in 1940, Newton increased his workload to protect his family and aid Japanese Americans to the detriment of his health and eyesight. He again worked day and night to preserve his company against union boycotts and hostile investor takeovers. In good times and in bad, he applied himself to forward looking tasks to steady situations and moved ahead.

In the early 1970s, Newton partnered with Antero Partanen and Osmo Paivinen to establish Wesley-Jessen of Scandinavia in Helsinki, Finland. This relationship created a partnership with Instrumentarium Oy (Ltd), an optical and medical supplier. Newton wanted to have a European representative to coordinate operations that were becoming too detailed and complex for him to handle along with his other WJ duties. He began a search for the coordinator using Bertil Olsen, management consultants in Stockholm. Among the potential candidates was Sandra Morgan from London, England. However, since she lacked skills in two foreign languages beyond English, she wasn't qualified for the position. Newton felt she had other relevant attributes and asked that Sandra be included among the interviews of eight potential candidates. Newton noted that,

At the end of the day, Sandra and I compared notes; they were identical in our impressions of the eight. I could not believe it. None fitted the bill, so we told Mr. Teague and Mr. Olsen. At that time, Mr. Teague said, "It is obvious that Sandra can fill the bill. Why don't you hire her for your representative in Europe?" ... We went on to Helsinki. After signing the agreement with Instrumentarium, our new partners in a new venture, while discussing the future of the company, Sandra and I had a few minutes to talk with Mr. Aulis Hauhia, the president of Instrumentarium. I began to realize that Sandra had a good grasp of the knowledge of people. She was bright, intelligent, caught on quickly, and seems to have an instinct for the proper decisions. (Wesley, 1988, pp. 178-179)

There was more than just praise for a talented young associate in Newton's words about Sandra. Sandra worked on a project to re-open the London office for WJ after John de Carle left to create his extended wear soft lens, the Permalens. In 1972, Newton and WJ President Orrin Stine agreed to bring Sandra to Chicago to do executive training for the European representative position. Roy Wesley helped Sandra locate suitable apartments in Chicago to rent for her stay in early January 1973. Following Cecilia's death and mourning period, some friends provided suggestions for potential marriage partners, but Newton wrote:

I thought, "I know just the person with whom I would like to live out the rest of my life." One day, after a particularly bad day, I took Sandra Morgan to dinner. She was training in Chicago at that time for the European position. I popped the question. The answer came back, "Yes." However, I would have to to to to Ireland where her father and mother had retired. (Wesley, 1988, p. 184)

Newton and Sandra went to Ireland and received permission from her parents to marry. At age 57, Newton married Sandra Morgan to begin a new life and family. They had five children: Morgan, Shona, twins (Justine and Jenna), and Taylor. After many years of resisting buyout offers for the company, Newton agreed to sell Wesley-Jessen in 1980. If anyone asked why he decided to sell at that time, he cryptically answered, "The birth of the twins made me sell."

Schering-Plough Pharmaceutical Company of New Jersey purchased Wesley-Jessen on September 23,1980. On the morning of the electronic transfer of funds, Newton, Lee, and Roy Wesley sat around the board of directors table with Orrin Stine, Irwin Panter, and others in the Green Room at the top of the Chicago Board of Trade building. In near silence, lost in thoughts, they waited for the moment when the money reached the Wesley-Jessen bank account. It was a strange experience anticipating an unseen life changing event heralded by a phone ringing and a voice confirming the arrival.

Expansion of space and workforce accompanied the sale. Wesley-Jessen moved from the seven floors at 37 S. Wabash to 128,000 square feet in Chicago's River North area at 400 W. Superior Street. The 600 employees were retained and augmented to 1,000. After a $13 million renovation, the grand opening was held in 1985 with Mayor Harold Washington officiating at the ribbon cutting ceremony. Later that year, Mayor Washington spoke at the Television Academy Luncheon saying,

> Chicago's story of revitalization of the last several years may best be told by the Wesley-Jessen contact lens company. An old Chicago-based firm, they are the leading manufacturer of contact lenses in the Midwest. They had outgrown their old factory and were ready to make a move. They looked around, considering other cities and other locales outside Chicago. But when they finally made their decision, they instead moved to another Chicago location, with plans to double their work force—symbolizing not only their own faith in Chicago, but a citywide renaissance. (Wesley, 1988, p. 110)

Wesley-Jessen continued to grow and went through several stages of further buy-outs and mergers through the years. To use Andy Warhol's expression, WJ had its 15 minutes of fame when Jon Stewart featured the company on *The Daily Show*. During Mitt Romney's 2012 Presidential campaign, he touted his business experience in turning Wesley-Jessen around and making a $300 million profit from a $6 million initial investment. Jon Stewart lampooned Romney and identified the company:

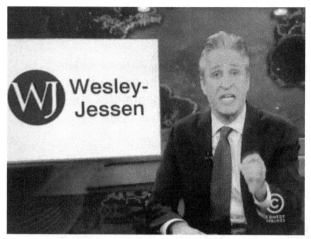

Jon Stewart on "The Daily Show," 1995.

Newton did not retire from working but continued his life-long interest in the eye care profession by continuing the work and educational seminars of NERF. Schering-Plough, the new owner of Wesley-Jessen, was not interested in keeping the Foundation as part of the company. Newton wanted to keep his favorite charity going so he retained all rights and assets of NERF. Newton and Sandra moved to a home in Northbrook, Illinois, a suburb to the north of Chicago to raise their family. NERF offices were located a mile and a half to the north of his home in Northbrook. After the passing of his brother, Edward Uyesugi, in Paoli, Indiana, Newton moved his brother's low vision contact lens practice to the NERF headquarters. Newton re-established a clinic to service the patients Dr. Uyesugi left behind and bring in new patients using his brother's techniques. Newton also created a new business, American Interprofessional Associates (AIA). AIA assisted doctors desiring retirement and the turn over of their practice to others. Newton continued to work until 2005, when he began to slow down. Newton died at the age of 93 in 2011.

Dr. Newton K. Wesley's life work and legacy made invisible contact lenses visible and present worldwide.

Dr. Newton K. Wesley's son, N. Lee Wesley, summarized his father's endeavors in a poem titled "Contacts" at the time of his death in 2011.

Contacts
Lee Wesley

You are the inventor of the first successful contact lens.
　　You were lying on a white-sheeted bed going blind,
　　Seeing two hundred starry images in your left eye,
　　and four hundred in your right.

I wonder how you could study for Earlham Indiana's pre-med exams,
　　With your Japanese-American wife and two baby boys languishing
　　In Minidoka, Idaho, in a sun-scorched camp surrounded by barbed-wire
　　And a rifle-laden guardhouse waiting for the war to end.

Were you too busy running in circles in Chicago
　　Where doctor after doctor told you it was hopeless?
　　Some said they don't know what to make of your condition,
　　Others said your eyes would rupture like volcanoes
　　And you would descend into a black starless night.

But one doctor said, "There is a miracle cure.
　　I'll put white plaster on your eyes,
　　To cast an impression of their shape,
　　So quarter-size pieces of shiny plastic can be molded
　　To fit on your brown eyes and under your lids."

This so-called miracle cure required
　　Bathing the lenses in a tear-like solution
　　And after seeing for a short time,
　　You find your eyes burning like fire.

So in a small Chicago basement, you and your partner
　　invented another lens, lighter, smaller,
　　Based on eye measurements from an instrument
　　That looked like a black Tommy gun.
　　Instead of white plaster, it shot light rays.

You cured your blindness with this small jewel of a lens.
　　And amazement after amazement
　　You wear this unnamed thing all day without pain.
　　You reason if you can, anyone can.

So like rock and roll stars criss-crossing the nation
　　Spreading the gospel of rock and roll.
　　You, in your single-engine plane,
　　Sputtered across the nation into city after city.

You spoke to newspapers, radio and TV stations
　　About contact lenses during the day.
　　You taught curious doctors how to fit them
　　At meetings during the night.
　　You said your goal was to put the word "contact
　　Lenses" in the dictionary.

And as you lie on a white hospital bed
　　With white shock of hair and white bushy sideburns.
　　I dread to hear the final call:
　　"The inventor of contacts has left the hospital–
　　Dr. Newton K. Wesley"

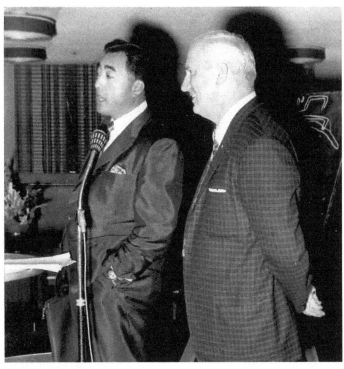

Newton Wesley and George Jessen, c. 1970. (Roy Wesley personal collection)

REFERENCES

Unless otherwise noted, quotations from Newton K. Wesley in the text are from his unpublished autiobiograpy manuscript or from his publishing autobiography, *Contacts–One Hundred Years Plus*.

Austin, Allan. "National Japanese American Student Relocation Council." Densho Encyclopedia. https://encyclopedia.densho.org National%20 Japanese%20American%20Student%20Relocation%20Council.

Bailey, Neal. "Neal Bailey's Contact Lens Chronicle." *Contact Lens Spectrum* 2 (1987): 2-64.

Baker, George N. Letter to President Willam Dennis, September 20, 1942.Earlham College Archives, EC V.05: Presidential Papers: William Cullen Dennis.

Beacher, L. Lester, *Contact Lens Technique*. New York: Beacher, 1941.

Bennett E.S., and B.A. Weissman, eds. *Clinical Contact Lens Practice*. Philadelphia: Lippincott Williams & Wilkins, 2005.

Bowden, Tim, and Andrew Gasson. "The Overseas Pioneers," *Contact Lens History*. British Contact Lens Association Monograph, 2006.

Bowden, Timothy J. *Contact Lenses. The Story.* London: Bower House, 2009.

Carr, B.J., and W. K. Stell. "The Science Behind Myopia." In *Webvision: The Organization of the Retina and Visual System*, editing by H. Kolb, E. Fernandez, annd R. Nelson. Salt Lake City (UT): University of Utah Health Sciences Center; 1995-. https://www.ncbi.nlm.nih.gov/books/ NBK470669/

Departments of Labor, Health, Education, and Welfare Appropriations for 1961. *Hearings before the Subcommittee of the Committee on Appropriations, House of Representatives*. 86 Congress, 2nd Sess., FDA Press Release HEW-J99. Washington, DC: Government Printing Office, 1961.

149

Dickinson, Frank. "Fourth International Congress of Contact Lens Practitioners, Munich, August 23-27, 1957." *The Optician*, (1957): 299-303.

Dickinson, F. "The value of micro-corneal lenses in progressive myopia," *The Optician*, (1957): 263–264.

"Edgewater Beach meeting," *Contacto* 3, no. 5 (1959): 131.

Feinbloom, William. "The Practice of Fitting Contact Lenses." *Journal of the American Optometric Association*, (1941): 1-46. https://hdl.handle.net/2027/osu.32436000139962

Fick, A.E. "Ein neues optisches Hilfsmittel bei unregelmässigem Astigmatismus." *Archiv für Augenhilk*, XVIII (1888).

Fick, A.E. "A contact lens," (trans. C. H. May). *Arch. Ophthalmol.* 19, (1888): 215–226.

Gasson, Andrew. "Overseas Contact Lens Pioneers." 2017. https://www.andrewgasson.co.uk/overseas-contact-lens-pioneers/

Goldberg, Joe B. "Long-term Effects of Contact Lens Wear." *Contact Lens Spectrum,* (June 2003). https://www.clspectrum.com/issues/2003/june-2003/readers-forum

Goss, David. "A History of Some Optometric Periodicals, Part 3." *Contact Lens Spectrum* 49, no. 3 (2018): 52.

"Growth of Oregon College." *The Optical Journal and Review*, (May 10, 1923): 53.

Hamm, Thomas D. "The Friends Collection at Earlham College," *The Library Quarterly: Information, Community, Policy* 60, no. 2 (1990), 139-149. https://doi.org/10.1086/602208

Harris, Donald H. "Myopia Control Now," *Orthokeratology* 3, (1976): 31-33.

Herguth, Robert. "$1 Million Dress Is Something to See." *Chicago Daily News*, July 29, 1959.

Jessen, George. Letter of Resignation, April 25, 1969. Roy Wesley personal letter collection.

Kaltenborn, H.V. "Broadcast of the bombing of Pearl Harbor, NBC radio report," December 7, 1941. https://www.youtube.com/watch?v=6muWK4VMbEI

Lamb, Jacqueline and Tim Bowden. "The History of Contact Lenses." In *Contact Lenses*, edited by Anthony Phillips and Lynne Speedwell, 2-17, New York: Elsevier, 2017.

Lloyd, Jack. "At 76, Phyllis Diller stakes out the comedy circuit." *The Baltimore Sun*, December 24, 1993.

Mandell, R.B. *Contact Lens Practice*. Springfield, IL. Charles C Thomas, 1998.

Mountford, John, David Ruston, and Trusit Dave. *Orthokeratology, Principles and Practice*. London: Butterworth-Heinemann, 2004.

Müller, A. *Brillengläser und Hornhautlinsen*. Inaugural Dissertation, University of Kiel, 1889.

Müller, F.E. *Ueber die Korrektion des Keratokonus und anderer Brechungsanomalien des Auges mit Müllers-chen Kontaktschalen*. Dissertation, University of Marburg, 1920.

Müller-Welt, A. "The Müller-Welt fluidless contact lens." *Optom. Wkly.* 41, (1950): 831–834.

Murray, George. "It Takes Work to Be Best." *The Chicago American*, July 13, 1959.

National Defense Migration: Hearings Before the United States House Select Committee Investigating National Defense Migration. 77th Congress, 2nd Sess., on February 26, 28, March 2, 1942, Part 30, "Portland and Seattle Hearings: Problems of Evacuation of Enemy Aliens and Others From Prohibited Military Zones." Washington, DC: Government Printing Office, 1942: 1-641.

National Student Relocation Council, Report of Progress, July 25, 1942. Earlham College Archives, EC V.05: Presidential Papers: William Cullen Dennis.

Nolan, Joseph. "The first meeting of the International Orthokeratology Society," *Contacto* 38, no. 4 (1995): 9-14.

Pearson, R.M."Karl Otto Himmler, manufacturer of the first contact lens." *Contact Lens & Anterior Eye* 30, (2007): 11-16.
Portland City Directory. City of Portland, 1939.

Reeves, Richard. *Infamy: The Shocking Story of the Japanese American Internment in World War II*. New York: Henry Holt and Company, 2015.

Shirrell, Elmer L.. Letter to Mrs. Cecilia K. Wesley, June 8, 1943. National Archives Building, Washington, DC, WRA Restricted Files, Stack 18W3, Row 10, Compartment 5.

Special Committee on Aging, Hearings before the Subcommittee on Frauds and Misrepresentations Affecting the Elderly. 88th Congress, 2nd Sess., Part 4B (Eye Care). Washington, DC: Government Printing Office, April 6, 1964: 413-430.

Swarbrick, Helen A. "Orthokeratology Review and Update." *Clin Exp Optom*. 89, no. 3 (2006): 124-43.

Townsley Malcom. "New equipment and methods for determining the contour of the human cornea." *Contacto* 11, (1967): 72.

Uyesugi, Newton. Letter to Governor Sprague, May 19, 1942, Oregon State Archives, Box 5, Folder 1.

Uyesugi, Newton. Letter to President Willam Dennis, April 12, 1942. Earlham College Archives, EC V.05: Presidential Papers: William Cullen Dennis.

Westport, Oregon History. http://pnwphotoblog.com/westport-oregon-history/

Wesley, Cecilia K. Letter to Elmer Shirrrell, June 2, 1943, National Archives Building, Washington, DC, WRA Restricted Files, Stack 18W3, Row 10, Compartment 5.

Wesley, Newton K. Autobiography. (unpublished manuscript n.d.) typescript, Roy Wesley personal collection.

———, Newton K. Scrapbook of Newton K. Wesley, c. 1937. Roy Wesley personal collection.

———, Newton K. Telephone Address Books, 1938-1950. Roy Wesley personal collection.

———, Newton K. Chapel Talk, January 22, 1943. Earlham College Archives, Presidential Papers: William Cullen Dennis.

———, Newton K. The Planning Committee, Wesley-Jessen Memorandum, 1970. Roy Wesley personal collection.

———, Newton K. *Contacts–One Hundred Years Plus*. Chicago: Vantage Press, 1988.

———, Newton K. Letter to Alice Shoji, March 6, 1989. Roy Wesley personal collection.

———, Newton K., and George N. Jessen. *Contact Lens Practice*. Chicago: Professional Press, 1953.

Wilson, Kermit. Letters, 1941-42. Roy Wesley personal collection.

APPENDIX

Wesley-Jessen Timeline and Locations

Newton Wesley went from basement research to founding a company at the end of World War II. Newton and George worked for 3 years (1944-1946) in the basement at 5218 N. Kenmore Ave., Chicago (photo in Chapter 6) making molded plastic scleral lenses and miniaturizing them into smaller lenses using "a lathe, drill press, grinding equipment, and dental molding equipment." They used a treadle sewing machine converted into a simple lathe. In 1946 the determined duo moved their primitive operation and the first contact lens radius cutting lathe designed by engineer Jim Kawabata into the office building where George and Newton had established their optometric specialty practice, the American Vision Center (1945).

1944 5218 N. Kenmore, basement research lab - 1944, George Jessen, Val Kuehn, and Newton Wesley.

1945 George Jessen and Newton Wesley established the American Vision Training Center as a specialty optometric practice. In the evenings, they trained new optometry school graduates in post-graduate courses at their American Optometric Center using the clinic facility in the Mallers Building.

1946 Mallers Building, 59 E. Madison St and 5 S Wabash Ave, Chicago. Established the Plastic Contact Lens Company to manufacture small corneal "microlens" Feb 13, 1946.

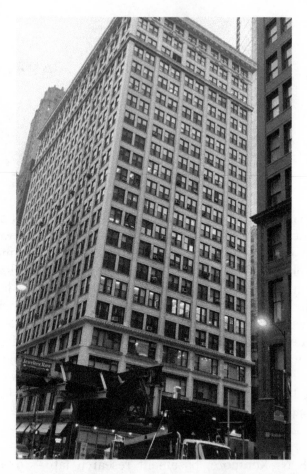

The Mallers Building at the corner of Madison and Wabash, Chicago, Illinois. Designed by Christian A. Eckstorm in 1910. Dr. Wesley occupied rooms on the 4th floor and the Jessen Wesley Clinic was on the 6th floor. (Roy Wesley personal collection)

1948 June 25, incorporation of The Plastic Contact Lens Company.

1952 Development of the "Sphercon" lens.

1956 Dr. Wesley established the National Eye Research Foundation. Oct 10, 1956 NERF incorporated as a non-profit, with The Fund of NERF as a 501(c)3 charitable.

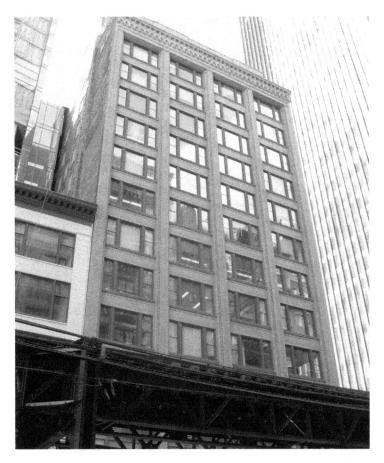

37 S. Wabash, Chicago. The Champlain building built 1902 by Holabird and Roche. The noted architect Ludwig Mies van der Rohe has his private office in the building. Wesley-Jessen occupied 7 of the 13 floors in the building. Manufacturing lab was on the 9th floor. (Roy Wesley personal collection)

1958 37 S. Wabash Ave, The Champlain Building

1961 Gage Building, 18 S. Michigan Ave (NKW Office, 6th floor with Japanese side room). Sweeping views of Grant Park and Lake Michigan.

1971 Wichterle and B&L launched soft contact lens in United States.

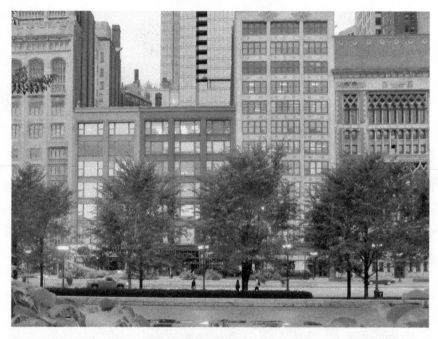

18 S. Michigan Avenue, Chicago (tall white building right of center). Newton's office was on the 6th floor facing Grant Park. NERF and Contacto offices were on the 9th floor. Three Gage Group Buildings in the center were built from 1890–1899 by Holabird and Roche with the façade of 18 S. Michigan designed by Louis Sullivan. (Roy Wesley personal collection)

1971 WJ has 27 US Offices with 4 Foreign (Buenos Aires, Argentina; Toronto, Ontario, Canada; Mexico City; Bogota, Columbia). By 1974, Affiliate foreign offices were also in Argentina (Buenos Aires, Cordoba, La Plata, Mar Del Plata, Mendoza Erwin Voss); Canada: Calgaray, Edmonton, Halifax, Montreal, Quebec, Saskatchewan, Toronto, Vancouver, and Winnipeg; Columbia, Bogota; Finland, Helsinki; Mexico (Gaudalajara, Mexico City); Peru, Lima; Uruguay, Montevideo.

1979 Introduction of Rigid Gas Permeable lenses (RGP)

1980 September 23, 1980. WJ sale to Schering-Plough, NJ.

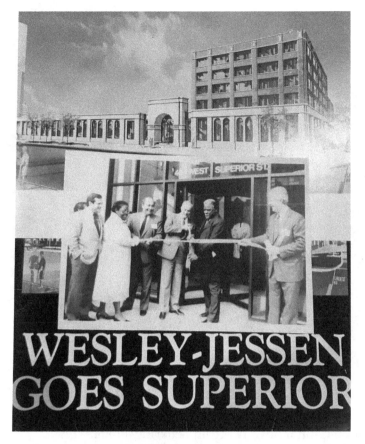

Mayor Washington was mayor of Chicago 1983-1987. The renovated building covered one large city block and was a former candy factory in the River North district of Chicago. Tax incentives were provided for WJ to move operations to the building with manufacturing on the first level and administration in the adjacent 5 story tower building. Employee growth from 400 to 1,100 employees. (Wesley-Jessen press release brochure, 1985)

1985 400 W. Superior St., Chicago. Mayor Harold Washington cut the ribbon for the Grand Opening ceremony.

1987 DuraSoft Colors sales up to $95 million.

1991 333 Howard St., Des Plaines, IL, 1991 - 2014.

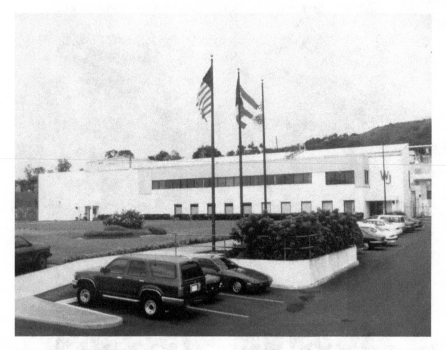

Wesley-Jessen Des Plaines, Illinois. 17-acre facility opened December 17, 1991. (Roy Wesley personal collection)

1995 Bain Capital buys WJ from Schering-Plough for $47 Million.

2001 Ciba Geigy buys WJ from Bain for $303 Million, 2,600 employees. Wesley-Jessen VisionCare merged with CIBA Vision.

2014 Alcon Ciba Vision, Fort Worth, TX (Freshlook Colors).

Wesley-Jessen Incorporations

PCL/WJ Anniversary Feb 13, 1946 according to Newton Wesley in "World of WJ, February 1970".

...

The Plastic Contact Lens Company, Incorporated June 25, 1948, Cert No 20876, IL Corp. (5 S Wabash Ave, Chicago)

Wesley-Jessen Contact Lens Co., Inc October 26, 1956. (5 S Wabash Ave, Chicago)

...

WJ Affiliate Branch Offices Incorporation Dates

United States

Atlanta, GA	Oct 8, 1959, Paul Williams, district manager
Boston, MA	August 12, 1960
Dallas, TX	May 28, 1959
Denver, CO	August 20, 1959, Merle Moebus, Branch Manager
Miami, FL	August 9,1960, Larry Miller, Office Manager
Milwaukee, WI	July 25, 1960
Minneapolis, MN	August 5, 1960
New Orleans, LA	August 9, 1960
New York, NY	Nov 19, 1959
Philadelphia, PA	August 9, 1960
Pittsburgh, PA	October 8, 1959
Portland, OR	July 25, 1960
St. Louis, MO	March 10, 1960, Harold Kuhlman, Branch Manager; Harvey Kopsky, Sales rep; Rena Atteberry, Secretary; Charles Johnson, lab technician.
San Francisco, CA	October 29, 1960
Seattle, WA	October 23, 1960

Foreign Distributorships

Mexico Exclusive	Victor Chiquiar-Arias
Bogoto, Columbia	Dr. Hernando Henao
Ponce de Leon, Puerto Rico	Dr. William J. Denton
Athens, Greece	Mrs. Berice Magoulas Papadiamantotoulos

···

EYE RESEARCH FOUNDATION, Inc. October 10, 1956, Illinois. Cert No 6933. (37 S. Wabash Ave, Chicago)

> Fund of The Eye Research Foundation, 501(c)3 non-profit
> July 6, 1959
>> Advisory Board
>> Leonard Bronstein, OD, Executive Secretary, Chicago
>> Ricardo Arruga,MD, Barcelona, Spain
>> Gilberto Cepero, MD, Havana, Cuba
>> Victor Chiquiar-Arias, OD, Mexico D.F., Mexico
>> Frank Dickinson, FBOA, St. Annes-on-Sea, England
>> Prof R Dudgagne, Paris, France
>> Tutomu Sato, MD, Tokyo, Japan
>> Wilhelm P. Soenges, DOS, Munich, Germany
>> Erwin Voss, OD, Buenos Aires, Argentina

···

Manufacturing
> Joseph Cinefro, first lab manager, then WJ Vice-President
> Kurt Wehking, Lab superintendant

···

WJ Consultation Department
> C. Robert Parker, OD, became Director of Consultation, Chicago Sales Manager, then National Accounts service manager. Oversaw domestic and overseas accounts. (Ref: World of WJ 1970)
> Art Hogan, OD

Carole Schwartz, OD
Brenice Ligman, OD

...

Research
   Malcolm Townsley, PhD
   Malcolm Bibby OD
   Alan Tomlinson, OD PhD
   Shah Chen, PhD

Marketing/Public Relations
   William Boyd
   Pat Morrisey

...

Miscellaneous Wesley-Jessen incorporations

Kolograph Corporation, Name changed to National Sound Projector Corp. Incorporated Feb 28, 1949; Dissolved in bankruptcy, May 27, 1954.

Quality Screw Machine Co., Organized October 15, 1951. Merged with National Sound Projector Corp., March 1953

San Incorporated, Jan 8, 1959. President Wolfram J. Dochterman, Formerly incorporated as Research Films, Inc., Jan 8, 1959.

TAMA, Inc. 30 E. Adams St. Chicago. July 27, 1957 incorporation date. Formerly incorporated as Chicago Visual Products Inc., name change to Opco Supplies, name change to Tama Inc.
   Pres: Bette Bagnell, Sec: Julian Anderson.
   Asst Sec: Emma Janies,
   Exec VP: John Graf
   Treasurer: William McGovern

The Contact Lens Publishing Company, Inc Nov 25, 1959.
(5 S Wabash Ave Chicago)

Foreign Offices

Foreign distributorships were established in the following countries:

Argentina
>Plastic Contact Lens of Argentina
>Dr. Erwin Voss
>Av. Pte. Roque S., Pena 720
>1035 Buenos Aires, Argentina

Brazil
>Pupilente-Wesley, S.A.
>Claus Dahns, General Manager
>Baixa Postal 45317
>Sao Paulo, Brasil

Canada
>Plastic Contact Lens Canada, Ltd.
>J.E. Casson
>21 Dundas Square, Suite 504
>Toronto, Ontario, M58 1B7
>Canada

>Imperial Contact Lens, Joint Venture
>Samuel Nisenboim

Columbia
>Dr. Hernando Henao
>Bogata, Columbia
>Barraquer Eye Institute Joint Venture

England (July 18, 1959)
>The Sphercon Contact Lens Company, Limited,
>John de Carle
>65 Grosvenor Street
>London W1, England.
>Mayfair 4331

Finland
>Wesley-Jessen of Scandinavia Oy
>Anteror Partanen, Osmo Paivinen
>Fl 357
>Aleksanterinkatu 15 B
>00100 Helsinki 10
>Finland

Greece
>Optical Papdiamantopoulos, Distributor
>Mrs. Beatrice Magoulas Papdiamantopoulos
>Athens, Greece

Mexico
>Plastic Contact Lens de Mexico
>Dr. Victor Chiquiar Arias
>Insurgentes Sur 107
>Mexico 6, D.F.

Ponce de Leon, Puerto Rico, Dr. William J. Denton

NERF National and World Congresses
Dr. Wesley International Meetings and Seminars

Year	Event
1956	Hawaii Optometric Association, Dr. Wesley Featured Guest Speaker and Honoree. Reef Hotel, Honolulu, Hawaii. February 1956.
	3rd International Society of Contact Lens Specialists Meeting (ISCLS), Urfarhn, Bavaria, Germany. August 1956. Dr. Wesley's first invitation to participate.
1957	4th International Society of Contact Lens Specialists Meeting (ISCLS), Urfarhn, Bavaria, Germany. August 1957.
	2nd National NERF Congress. November, 1957 NY, Chicago, Los Angeles. (*Contacto*, Vol II, No. 1, January 1958)
1958	3rd National NERF CL Congress. November.
1959	National CL Congress. 4th national became the **1st world NERF CL congress**. Aug 2-4. Edgewater Beach Hotel in Chicago, Illinois. (*Contacto* March, 1959)
1960	Fourth Japanese Contact Lens Congress. June 26, at Nagoya, Japan. (*Contacto* October, 1960, p. 469)
	5th National Contact Lens Congresses (*Contacto* January 1960) Oct 30-31. Biltmore Hotel, New York City Nov 13-14. Sheraton Towers, Chicago Nov 20-21. Jack Tar Hotel, San Francisco
1961	Contact Lens Research Conference. July 17-18. Stardust Hotel, Las Vegas.
1962	6th National Contact Lens Congress, 1962. Nov 12-14, 1961. Sherman Hotel, Chicago. (*Contacto* April, 1961, p. 149)
	7th National Contact Lens Congress. Oct 14-16. LaSalle Hotel, Chicago. (*Contacto* February, 1962, p. 41) *Contacto* Nov. 1962

1963	2nd World NERF Contact Lens Congress. August 4-6. Edgewater Beach Hotel, Chicago, Illinois.
1964	Contact lens meetings, Erwin Voss, Argentina. Meeting with President Umberto A. Illia of Argentina in the President's Pink House with Dr. Erwin Voss and Dr. Liberatore. Press coverage in Spanish, German, and English. Feb 12-13, Buenos Aires, Argentina.

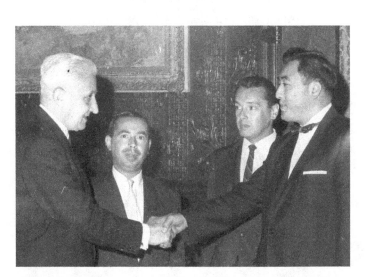

Left to right: Argentina President Illia, Dr. Erwin Voss, Dr. Libertore, Dr. Newton Wesley, February 13, 1964, President's Pink House, Buenos Aires. (Roy Wesley personal collection)

	9th National NERF Contact Lens Congress. November 15-17. Hotel Continental, Chicago. (*Contacto*, March, 1964, p. 19)
1965	Hotel Ginrinsou, Otaru-shi, Hokkaido Meeting, June 4.
	Ryuguden Hotel, Hakone Meeting, June 1965; Enoshima Kanko Hotel, Okinawa

Contact Lens Society Japan, Meeting in Tokyo.
President: Prof. Yasuharu Kuwabara.
Dr. Newton K. Wesley (America) *Ambulatory Method of Contact Lens Fitting*, June 1965, Tokyo.

10th National NERF Contact Lens Congress.
November 7-9, 1965, Ambassador Hotels, Chicago.
(*Contacto*, June, 1965, p. 6)

1966   12th ISCLS, Xochimilco, Mexico, April.

Anchorage, Alaska. Alaska Optometric Association invited guest speaker. June 8.

Newton Wesley prepartory trip to Athens, Greece to set up meetings. Visit with Beatrice Margoulis. September 19.

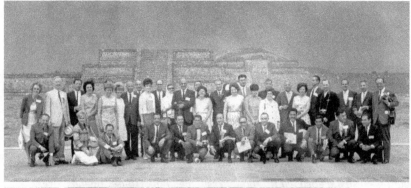

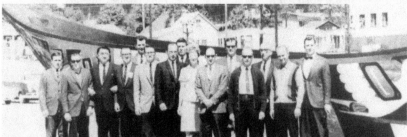

TOP: 12th ISCLS visit to Aztec temples at Teotihuacan, Mexico, April 1966. Newton Wesley front row, second from right. BOTTOM: Alaska Optometric Association Meeting, June 6. 1966. Anchorage, Alaska. Newton Wesley third from left. (Roy Wesley personal collection)

Hong Kong, China, Contact Lens Meeting, Tai Pak (Floating Palace) Restaurant. September 23.

1967   14th International Society of Contact Lens Specialists Meeting (ISCLS), Athens, Greece. September 6-13. NERF reported with a special hardbound *Contacto*.

Hong Kong Contact Lens Meeting, Sea Palace, Hong Kong, China. September 19.

Philippine Contact Lens Association, Manila, Philippines. The Plaza Convention Hall, September 24. Dr. Wesley invited Guest Speaker.

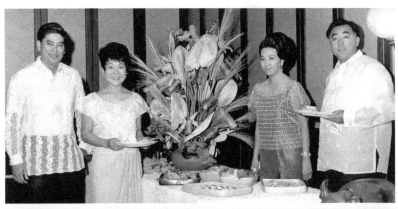

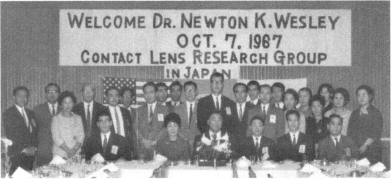

TOP: Dr. Gamahil M. Gonzalez, Mrs. Cecilia Wesley, Mrs. Gonzalez, Dr. Newton K. Wesley, Manilla, Philippines, September 24, 1967. BOTTOM: Contact Lens Research Group in Japan, Honored Guest Lecturer. October 7, 1967. (Roy Wesley personal collection)

12th National NERF CL Congress (*Contacto*
September, 1967, p. 7)
  Nov 5-6. Sheraton Plaza, Boston
  Nov 13-14. Caesar's Palace, Las Vegas
  Nov 19-20. Palmer House, Chicago

1968   3rd World NERF Contact Lens Congress, Palmer
House, Chicago, August 1968.

Japan Ophthalmological Society. Dr. Wesley guest
speaker. October 1968. Hiroshima, Japan.

1969   ISCLS Bermuda Meeting, Castle Club, Castle
Harbour Hotel (now Tucker's Point Hotel),
Bermuda. August 25-29.

Newton Meeting in Tokyo, Japan. October 1969.

1970   April 4-6. Nassau. Bahamas

April 11-13. Pittsburgh

XXI Congresso Internacional Oftalmologia, Rio de
Janeiro, Brazil. May 1970.

14th National CL Congress (*Contacto* June, 1970,
pp. 44-49)
  Nov 15-17. Chicago
  Nov 22-24. Las Vegas

1971   15th National Contact Lens Congress (*Contacto*
June, 1973, p. 66)
  Nov 21-23. Las Vegas. (Bob Newhart)
  (*Contacto* Dec, 1972, pp. 24-31/ Sept, 1970, p.
  55./ March, 1971, pp. 58-59.)

16th National CL Congress Nov 7-10. Las Vegas
Sands Hotel (Sammy Davis, Jr.).

1972   4th NERF World Contact Lens Congress. July 14-
16. Tokyo, Japan. Imperial Hotel. (*Contacto* June,
1970, p. 67. / December, 1970, p. 42.)

1973   18th International NERF Congress. Aug 28-30,
1973. Buenos Aries, Argentina. (*Contacto* June,
1973, p. 2)

1974   Aug 10-12. International CL Congress co-sponsored
NERF+ CL Society of Great Britain,
Montreux, Switzerland.

Nov 17-21. 19th International NERF Congress Las Vegas.

1975   20th International Congress. Nov 16-24. Sahara Hotel in Las Vegas, then the Princess Hotel in Acapulco (*Contacto* January, 1976, pp. 24-28)

1976   Contact Lens Society Japan, Meeting in Osaka, Japan. President: Prof. Reizo Manabe (Osaka University). Dr. Newton K. Wesley presented the Memorial Lecture on Continuous Focal Lenses. June 1976.

Western Orthokeratology Section of NERF, educational seminar, Hyatt Lake Tahoe. June 19. (*Contacto*, Calendar of Events, May 1976, p. 1)

5th World CL Congress (NOT INTERNATIONAL. Nov 7-11, 1976. Sahara Hotel, Las Vegas (*Contacto* January, 1977, pp. 30-35)

1977   21st Congress. April 17-24, 1977. Bogata and Caracas (*Contacto* July, 1997. pp. 40-41.) (*Contacto* January, 1978, pp. 34-40)

May 5-19. NERF International Congress, Kyoto, Japan.

Newton receives Medical Research Degree from Osaka University Medical School, Osaka, Japan. May 22 (Showa 52).

Oct 29-Nov 4. International Congress. Ilitkai Hotel, Honolulu.

Nov 5-9. MGM Grand Hotel, Las Vegas.

1979   NERF Las Vegas, November 13.

Osaka, Japan November 20.

1980   NERF Symposia: March 16, Chicago; March 23, Milwaukee; April 20, St. Louis; April 27, Detroit. (*Contacto*, March 1980, p. 2)

National-International Contact Lens Congress, Regency-Hyatt Hotel, Chicago. May 31-June 1. (*Contacto*, May, 1980, p. 2)

25th Silver Jubilee International Contact Lens Congress, MGM Grand Hotel, Las Vegas, NV. October 26-30. (*Contacto*, March, 1980, p.2)

	November 30. Midwest Congress, Marriott Hotel, Chicago. (*Contacto*, May, 1980. p. 2)
1981	March 17-23. "Around The World," various cities including congresses co-sponsored with societies of Japan, the Philippines, India and other countries.
	June 6-7. National International Contact Lens Congress, Sheraton O'Hare, Chicago.
	July 1-August 26. Basic Update Course for international visitors. NERF and other optometric and ophthalmological institutions.
	September 26-27, Optifar/NERF, Continuing Education and Contact lens certification, Anaheim, California. (*Contacto*, September 1981, p. 41)
	November 16-19. 26th International Contact Lens Congrss, Nevada Dunes Hotel, Las Vegas, NV. (*Contacto*, January, 1981, p. 1)
1983	April 30-May 1. NERF National/International Contact Lens Congress, Sheraton-O'Hare, Chicago. (*Contacto*, July, 1983, p. 30).
	November 6-10. 28th International Contact Lens Congress, Caesars Palace, Las Vegas. Theme: "All of the Latest in Eye Care". (*Contacto* May, 1983, p. 1) Theme changed to "Set Your Sights on the Future in Eye Care." (*Contacto* July, 1983, p. 1)
1984	NERF/AIF 29th International Contact Lens Congress. Riviera Hotel, Las Vegas, NV. Octobr 31-November 4. (*Contacto:* Mini-Abstracts, August, 1984, p. 3)
1985	Winter 'Get Away' Meetings, AIF/NERF. Phoenix AZ January 27-28. Granada Royale Hometel, Phoenix. Orlando, FL Feb 28-March 1. Ramada Court of the Flags.
1987	32nd Annual Contact Lens Congress NERF/AIA October 15-18, The Frontier Hotel, Las Vegas, NV. (*Contacto*, Vol 1, No. 1, 1987, p. 3)
	Midwest Conference, Pheasant Run, St. Charles, IL May 15.

1988	Midwest Conference, Hotel Sofitel, O'Hare, Rosemont, IL May 15. (*Contacto,* 1988, p. 3)
	The Caribbean Course, August 15-24. Jamaica.
	33rd Annual Contact Lens Congress, Golden Nugget Hotel, Las Vegas, NV November 3-6. (*Contacto* 1988, p.3)
1989	35th Annual CL Congress. Oct 22-25,1990. Mirage Hotel, Las Vegas, NV. (*Contacto* 1989, #1&2, p. 58)
1991	36th Annual International CL Congress. Oct 14-17. Mirage Hotel, Las Vegas, NV. (*Contacto* 1990, #1&2, pg. 4)
1992	Annual International CL Congress and Continuing Education Program. Oct 4-8. Mirage Hotel, Las Vegas, NV.
1993	NERF'S Global Congress. July 16-18. (*Contacto* 1993, #1, p. 2)

Speech of Hon. EVERETT McKINLEY DIRKSEN of Illinois in the Senate of the United States, Wednesday, July 22, 1959. "The Contact Lens Industry" Congressional Record Proceedings and Debates of the 86th Congress, First Session.

The complete text of Senator Dirksen's speech, as published in the *Congressional Record,* is reproduced on the following pages.

(Not printed at Government expense)

Congressional Record

PROCEEDINGS AND DEBATES OF THE 86*th* CONGRESS, FIRST SESSION

The Contact Lens Industry

SPEECH

OF

Hon. EVERETT McKINLEY DIRKSEN

OF ILLINOIS

IN THE SENATE OF THE UNITED STATES

Wednesday, July 22, 1959

Mr. DIRKSEN. Mr. President, a good many years ago a young man in Chicago by the name of Dr. Newton K. Wesley was told he had an eye disease. Anyone who has ever had eye trouble becomes thoroughly sympathetic to that condition in someone else. Doctors told him the disease was incurable, and that he would go blind. So first he enrolled in a school for the blind. Second, he refused to believe the doctors, and started to see what could be done. He went all over the United States. The best clinicians told him some pressure had to be inserted on the eye. That could be done in the form of a contact lens. So he consulted with another doctor in Chicago by the name of George Jessen.

These two men set themselves to the business of research into this particular eye disease. Out of their research and out of their diligence, there came a great nourishment for the so-called contact lens industry. It has now gone so far that, insofar as I know, there are 15,000 contact lens practitioners in the country, and there are 77 laboratories devoted to research in that field. Every year they hold a congress. I think this coming year they are to hold a world congress.

519028—72000

All this has come about as the result of the efforts of a young man who was in danger of losing his sight. He refused to accept blindness as his inevitable fate. He set himself to a task and, by his efforts, he has enriched mankind. The results of his efforts involve not only improving the sight of millions of people, but enabling them to pursue professions, vocations, and avocations with greater facility and with greater efficiency, and his efforts have also resulted in improving the incomes of those whose eye deficiencies were thereby remedied.

In connection with these observations, Mr. President, I ask unanimous consent to have printed in the RECORD a statement by the Eye Research Foundation, which is a nonprofit organization located in Chicago, and dedicated exclusively to research into eyes and contact lenses.

There being no objection, the statement was ordered to be printed in the RECORD, as follows:

EYE RESEARCH FOUNDATION,
Chicago, Ill.

Hon. EVERETT M. DIRKSEN,
Senator from Illinois,
Senate Office Building, Washington, D.C.:

The Eye Research Foundation, headquartered in Chicago, Ill., is a nonprofit organization dedicated to the research of eyes and contact lenses exclusively. Founded 4 years ago in Chicago, the organization is truly international with members and committees functioning in more than 20 nations. We are justifiably proud of such growth in such a short period of time. Verily, Chicago has become the world leader in research and development of the contact lens.

2

To bring this about, the Eye Research Foundation sponsors a National Contact Lens Congress in three leading cities of the United States annually. At these meetings contact lens practitioners from all over the country—and some foreign countries—meet to exchange information and procedures as well as the latest techniques, developments and ideas in the contact lens field.

Marking the vast strides this industry has made over the past 4 years, in addition to the constant calls being made on the foundation by practitioners from foreign lands, the Eye Research Foundation is pleased to announce the First World Contact Lens Congress to be held in Chicago on August 2, 3, 4 of this year. Official invitations have gone out and replies have been received indicating that representatives of more than 20 nations will be in attendance.

The first world congress will be a quadrennial event.

It is the belief of the directors of the foundation that this single meeting will move the contact lens field many research years ahead, and will open areas of vision correction for millions of persons as a result of analysis which will be presented and adopted.

Beyond this single endeavor to broaden the ground for an international exchange of scientific thinking, the foundation is hopeful that the First World Contact Lens Congress will represent an important contribution to international efforts toward world peace. At a time when scientific fields are holding the attention of the world, the Eye Research Foundation, through this first world conclave, is contributing to peaceful and better existence.

Additionally, we feel that this First World Contact Lens Congress is of particular importance because in today's world of marked international tensions, a common council where representatives from all countries can meet in common conclave to exchange ideas, procedures, techniques and culture is very much to be desired. Let us hope that the time is not too far off when all of our goals—national as well as international—will be achieved, and our problems resolved by just such meetings conducted in peaceful friendship.

The Eye Research Foundation was established through the inspiration and energies of a single individual, Dr. Newton K. Wesley, of Chicago, who as a young man was faced with the prospect of eventual blindness through an unusual eye condition. After years of searching, his condition was arrested and vision restored through the miracle of contact lenses, with respect to which he has done phenomenal development and research. It was through this experience that he decided to devote his life to the advancement of the contact lens field.

In the 4 years since its founding the Eye Research Foundation has spearheaded the contact lens field to a point where it now represents surcease from suffering and even sight itself to many thousands who have restricted vision or would even be sightless.

In addition to improving the sight of many millions of persons through its research and development, the contact lens industry has greatly advanced the growth and incomes among the 38,000 members of the eye professions in our country and thousands more abroad.

The Eye Research Foundation was founded under the laws of the State of Illinois. Today its influence is felt throughout the world and its list of members and contributors number in the thousands.

The foundation organized the National Contact Lens Congresses which meet each November—officially designated as National Contact Lens Month—and which are attended by thousands of eye specialists.

The foundation also established an annual series of meetings called the research study group. This gathering is for the purpose of exposing exceptional contact lens research to leading figures in the field.

In addition, the foundation has encouraged and sponsored individual and group research; established fellowships to encourage further individual research; and has bestowed honors on those who have contributed exceptional and successful research to the contact lens field.

It is this spirit of interest and energy that aided growth of the number of contact lens practitioners in the United States to 15,000; and increased the contact lens laboratories in our country from 14 to 77; as well as having encouraged millions of persons to wear the tiny vision aids.

To further stimulate professional interest in the contact lens field, the foundation com-

519028—72000

3

municates to members of the eye professions through Contacto Journal, a monthly publication in which outstanding research and case histories are reported and read by 20,000 eye specialists.

The foundation also formed the first world referral and communication list, whereby professional persons in all countries are able to correspond with others conducting mutual research. This effort has fostered unselfish fellowship through the eye professions.

In its January 1958 issue, Contacto Journal printed a report on the Eye Research Foundation, its purpose, and its founder, Dr. Newton K. Wesley.

Contacto Journal noted that at the age of 21, Dr. Wesley was told he had an eye condition known as keratoconus. This strange malady had no known cure and in almost all cases led to ultimate blindness. On one hand Wesley accepted his fate and enrolled in a school for the blind, and on the other refused to believe the diagnosis.

For the next 4 years he traveled the entire United States, calling at every noted eye clinic, hospital, and eye specialist's office looking for a solution. In each case, he was told his condition was hopeless.

Only one solution, some said, would be a pressure bandage—a very special contact lens to arrest the progress of the disease. At this point, Dr. Newton K. Wesley met a Chicagoan, Dr. George Jessen, who had a basic interest and understanding of the principles behind contact lenses. Together they set out to make the contact lens which would save Wesley's eyesight. The two turned Jessen's basement into a laboratory and began a 6-year research. The program was carried on during holidays, evenings, and every spare moment. Many times, neither saw his family for days.

Finally, when Wesley's vision had regressed to elbow-length vision distance, the pair produced a contact lens which would not only arrest keratoconus, but could reshape the distorted window of the eye so that 20/20 vision was achieved instantly. Dr. Wesley has arrested an eye disease which afflicts thousands.

While Wesley's vision began to fail rapidly during those 6 years of research, he had a dream that someday he would be in a position to foster eye research so that others

519028—72000

would not be faced with personal research to save their own eyesight. And, today, the Eye Research Foundation is a reality.

In 1958 a board of directors was established as a beginning step. Prominent contact lens practitioners from all over the world lent their time and knowledge, and under this working group the first of the annual National Contact Lens Congresses was evolved and brought to a successful conclusion.

Early in 1957, Contacto Journal was set up as an official publication of the Eye Research Foundation. The aims of Contacto are simple. The contact lens field is growing to such proportions that it needs an organ of communication. New techniques, new processes of manufacturing, new methods of detection and treatment of ocular abnormalities are being achieved daily. Under the guidance of its editorial board of advisers, Contacto will provide an additional step toward achieving the humanitarian goals of the Eye Research Foundation. The publication is circulated widely throughout the world.

The formation of the Eye Research Foundation, the bylaws of which are printed herein, is a great step in our time toward solving the problems of those visually afflicted.

BYLAWS OF EYE RESEARCH FOUNDATION

Article I

Purposes

The purposes of the corporation as stated in its certificate of incorporation are: To encourage and aid research relating to the eye and contact lenses as a means to correct vision; to promote and foster education (not including the operation of a postsecondary educational institution or a vocational school) in the aforesaid fields by studying, exchanging, publicizing, and analyzing development, inventions, ideas, and concepts, by conducting seminars and conventions, by establishing scholarships, teaching chairs, and research programs in recognized schools, universities and other institutions, and by issuing publications of scientific and educational value relating to the eye and contact lenses as a means to correct vision.

The corporation also has such powers as are now or may hereafter be granted by the General Not-for-Profit Corporation Act of the State of Illinois.

U.S. GOVERNMENT PRINTING OFFICE: 1959

CPSIA information can be obtained
at www.ICGtesting.com
Printed in the USA
BVHW031334240621
610211BV00018B/2306/J

9 781945 398070